DNA Powered Health

*Unlock Your Potential
to Live with
Energy and Ease*

by **SHERIDAN GENRICH**

Praise for *DNA Powered Health*

'For so many of us, life's traumatic events can impact our minds and our bodies in ways we may never have imagined. Such events can lock in epigenetic changes that can have long-term effects on both our physical and mental health. In *DNA Powered Health*, Sheridan has drawn on her own personal health experiences, coupling these with extensive clinical expertise in nutrition, nutrigenomics and lifestyle medicine. The result? A practical approach you can use to identify and unravel the 'blocks' that have prevented your recovery. *DNA Powered Health* shows you how to take back control of your own health, systematically retraining your mind in overcoming the imbalances that have stolen your physical and mental health for so long.'
— *Dr Christine Houghton PhD.,BSc.,R.Nutr.*
   Nutritional Biochemist

"*DNA Powered Health* is a must-have comprehensive guide for anyone who's felt overwhelmed and unsafe in their bodies when faced with the reality of today's challenges. It gives one a 'superpower' to know ourselves and find the wisdom to change with confidence. A well-constructed and engaging read, this book is a road map for healing holistically by utilizing both ancestral and modern knowledge. It can help you refine and unlock your full health potential, so you can enjoy optimal health and live life to the fullest."
—*Dr Irina Antonova PhD,*
   Author & UQ Biotechnology Researcher

"Sheridan Genrich provides us with a very important conversation, one we all need to be having. Why do we respond differently to the events in our life? By understanding our genes, we understand who we are and how we respond to the world around us. Gaining these great insights about ourselves we can make the best possible decisions that will unlock a different kind of gene expression and change the cycle of stress, trauma and ill health. *DNA Powered Health*, provides an understanding of the worlds of genetics and epigenetics and how we can make daily choices to overcome our health challenges, both mental and physical."
— *Dr Yael Joffe, PhD Nutrigenomics RD (SA),*
   Author & Translational Genomics Expert

Disclaimer
While every effort has been made to ensure the accuracy of the
information in this book, it is not intended to replace professional medical advice. This book contains general information
and advice related to the potential benefits of using a food and
a lifestyle approach to improve individual health outcomes. The
author and publisher expressly disclaim responsibility for any
adverse effects that may result from the use or application of the
information contained in this book. A healthcare professional
should be consulted regarding your specific medical situation.

First edition
ISBN paperback: 978-0-6459623-0-7
ISBN e-book: 978-0-6459623-1-4

NATIONAL
LIBRARY
OF AUSTRALIA

A catalogue record for this
book is available from the
National Library of Australia

DEDICATION

To my grandmother
I was too young to relieve the suffering I watched you
endure with multiple sclerosis. Despite the autoimmune
attack on your brain, your kind heart and unwavering
faith in the divine kept your mind clear. Your spirit
sparked my desire to help others take care of their human
body in the limited time we have on this planet.

CONTENTS

Unexpected things happen, sometimes taking us to heights we'd never imagine possible.

How we handle these times of adversity is unique to each of us.

Imprints can be so deep in our memories that they change how we relate to ourselves and others.

As a highly sensitive person, I understand the challenges that come with feeling and sensing more energy in the environment.

I know what it's like to struggle and feel utterly hopeless.

Still, I've survived those hardest times. Scraping at the surface for me was years of sleep problems from jet lag in my work as a flight attendant, which played havoc on my emotional state and intimate relationships. Winning the genetic lottery was not my fate either. Autoimmunity, obesity and mental stress genes are all high risk for me.

I never gave up and kept searching for answers and new ways of thinking. I found the strength to take control of my present and future.

Truly, I believe every bit of that strength in me stems from my meditation practice of Falun Gong. Without it, I wouldn't exist as I am, nor would this book.

In 2001, I started this mind and body practice – also called Falun Dafa – at a local park. The qigong-style exercises gave me a positive outlook beyond what I'd previously known, by combining a way of living with the principles of truth, compassion and tolerance. I also rarely ever got sick, despite exposure to hundreds of people in my work life.

At the same time that I was experiencing the amazing health

benefits of Falun Gong, I learned about what was happening in China. Widespread popularity of Falun Gong rose in China when it was first introduced to the public in 1992. Chinese Communist Party (CCP) began a brutal campaign against it in 1999 when a huge crackdown was unleashed across the country. Practitioners were taken from their homes or workplaces and imprisoned, tortured, executed and even organ harvested if they did not renounce the spiritual practice.

I never imagined, as a Westerner, what could happen to me. That all changed when I landed in Beijing for a work stopover in late 2008.

My name was given to the onboard manager by the immigration officials who met the aircraft that night. My world was rocked by a call to my workstation instructing me to disembark the aircraft before the passengers. This never happened to any airline crew on landing. I had no reference point for facing this.

I quickly shifted into a hyper-alert state that I had never experienced before.

I remember thinking, "*Oh no. This is not good! Get me out of here!*"

My heart was pounding through my chest. I wanted to escape. Except there was nowhere to go.

Instead, there was the humiliation of walking to the entrance of the aircraft. I was acutely aware of the passengers and crew who were watching me being taken away.

Two stern-looking Chinese immigration officials met me at the aircraft door.

My gut tensed up when they took my passport off me. Although dressed in my Australian work uniform, I felt deeply exposed. My thoughts focused on finding support, *"who would come with me?"* But no one on my side came.

Chinese security escorted me past the brightly lit immigration lines and dispatched me into a darker private room. I was isolated from my colleagues. Alone with two foreign officials.

My whole body froze. Fully numb. I thought, *"how quickly has my night changed!"*

Asking myself, *is this what a "deer in headlights" feels like*?

An indescribable feeling of shock overcame me, like nothing I'd felt before. I felt a huge rush of adrenaline surge through my body and my muscles tensed.

In an unconscious attempt for my peace of mind, I tried to escape the reality of the situation. I disassociated from my body. I experienced a new level of what is described as a dysregulated nervous system. What I'd later learn was called a "freeze response".

After some time a different male uniformed official came and began interrogating me about my Chinese friends. They must have had me under surveillance for some years to know this much detail. The Chinese official's harsh tone and manner felt threatening and awkward. He told me that they were ordering a search of my check-in bags.

Tension in the room rose when he removed from my bag a spiritual book about Falun Gong – the teachings for how to live day-to-day life based on truth, compassion and tolerance. Official confiscation of my book was the catalyst for intense verbal abuse that followed. They were clearly targeting me for my spiritual faith.

After bombarding me with angry insults and abuse for quite some time, the Chinese officials eventually decided to send me back to Sydney. Further abuse and bullying behaviour from these officials followed as they escorted me onto the aircraft to be sent home as a passenger.

This scene caused me significant distress and embarrassment in front of my co-workers and business class passengers. It was like the Chinese authorities just continued to say and do whatever they wanted, without any formal legal basis given.

I was lucky to get out though. Others had been illegally incarcerated for years.

The sad part was that Chinese airport authorities couldn't see that they were victims too. Believing and following lies passed on from their country's leaders.

While completely exhausted, even delirious, I was relieved to arrive back home in Sydney. Although I soon found out that this wasn't the end of the drama.

I had not been charged, arrested, or even given any paperwork, to explain why I had been treated in such a way.

The airline did not report this to the governing bodies of Australia for a full investigation. I was stood down despite my exemplary work record spanning seven years with the airline. I felt disciplinary action was extreme. Shortly after they decided to terminate my international work contract.

This triggered me to initiate a legal process based on unfair dismissal.

Anything less would seem to be an admission of wrongdoing on my part.

Alone and unfamiliar with the Federal justice system, it was me against a big corporation with deep pockets. I didn't give up though.

I persisted when many others told me it was not worth it. For me, though the truth is a core traditional value that is always worth it.

Determined to seek justice I was fortunate to gain the support of a strong Sydney legal team (two barristers and a solicitor), who provided advice and representation.

Many months followed meeting with lawyers to prepare a case of unfair dismissal.

Later the following year that successful outcome eventuated. The judge ordered that I be reinstated to my former international employment status.

Throughout this time of life and legal event I thought I was coping well but in reality, I'd developed a habit of suppressing negative emotions which was affecting me physically. My body expressed what my mind could not.

The shock of that night in Beijing had deeply jolted my nervous system.

Reliving that event through the gruelling years that followed with legal action, kept my nervous system in full "survival mode".

I never considered that I held any stored trauma.
In persistent denial of any emotional effects, I kept telling myself, "*I am fine.*"

However there was so much disconnection going on within me. After all, it is not possible to think our way into feeling safe. Safety is a feeling that exists in the body first.

The daily exercise movements of Falun Dafa improved my sleep. Reading the teachings allowed me to trust, let go and endure more than I could've imagined.

I felt the spiritual connection supported my emotional and physical health. My faith was also instrumental in helping me get through this time without needing any medication.

To those who knew me, I was healthy, busy getting things done and had been functioning "normally." I had started my own health consulting business while flying part-time and raising a baby boy.

However, unknowingly my nervous system had been stuck in a trauma response since that frightful event in China. Unaware there was a connection between the China incident and ongoing vivid flashbacks. Accompanied by hyper-alertness and social withdrawal.

The toll on me had been huge emotionally, financially and physically.

The full impact and further personal challenges unfolded in my relationship in the years soon after.

I don't want my suffering to be for naught.

I've navigated through a whole process of loss and grief.

I've come through this with an open heart and a massive mission to help as many people as I can.

To help you recover from any unresolved trauma, with less struggle and more alignment in mind and body.

My message is of hope and to share with you what I've learned along the way through living the heart-centred principles of truth, compassion and tolerance.

I feel fortunate to have been on a learning quest for clinical and self-improvement for many years. This search helped me realise the need to understand tendencies within my unique DNA – all related to high sensitivities coming from changes in my blood sugars and nervous system. Addressing these impacted my overall hormone balance and was a foundational part of feeling emotionally stronger and more willing to socially reconnect.

Before this awakening and reset of my own, I struggled with relentless cravings, mood and energy swings. It felt endless, each day repeating itself, over and over.

In the afternoons I used to need a quick energy boost, leading me to overindulge in foods I thought would rejuvenate me. But inevitably, a crash would follow, leaving me feeling depleted and wanting to withdraw again.

This changed when I learned how to support my DNA through eating at regular meal times, choosing the right foods to balance my blood sugars, plenty of time in nature and daily meditation. Thankfully these strategies worked very quickly. They helped me more frequently feel calm, reduce cravings and keep my energy levels on an even keel. I began to again feel a sense of safety and trust within my mind and body. Feelings that had eluded me for years.

In different ways, most of us experience some degree of traumatic stress throughout life. I've heard from so many people in the clinic, like you, who experience this same endless cycle. I know that highly sensitive people can often struggle to return to their full potential. This inspired me to write this book and share my own successes and those I've worked with. I want to give you the awareness of these genetic tendencies and the actionable steps to balance your moods, blood sugar levels and if relevant, maintain sustainable weight loss without the struggles and disappointments of the next fad diet.

Best-selling author, Naval Ravikant stated,
"If you want to write a good book, you must first become the book."

So here it is!

It is my hope that the research in this book and my story of struggle and recovery will help you to become the best version of yourself.

Using an approach that addresses your genetic foundations can make for faster improvements and motivate you to stay on track. You will learn why specific body systems benefit from some methods or actions more than others, so you can choose to experiment with these as a priority for your healing.

Understanding and applying various lifestyle tools with a personalised health strategy can start today.

INTRODUCTION

No two people are alike. We are different in our experiences of trauma, genetic makeup, health history, lifestyles and family dynamics. Our ability to recover from adversity and avoid getting stuck in cycles of self-sabotage often stems from our thinking and behaviours.

In my clinical work, it is common to hear someone comment, "It feels like I'm always in "survival mode" and can't cope with more."

Can you relate? Do you often find yourself struggling to keep up with the competing demands of your career and home life?

Are you constantly on the run from one commitment to the next, compromising your own health and well-being in the process?

Maybe you're the person everyone calls on to fix things – you're usually the competent and confident person who still functions well, even when the pressure is high and time is scarce. But it's wearing you down and affecting your health – you aren't coping as well as you used to.

Living in survival mode with unresolved stress exhausts both our mental and physical resources. You might call it feeling overwhelmed, adverse or chronically stressed. I'm not talking about the everyday pressures, but an accumulation of too much pressure over many months or years.

Eventually, this leads you to feel you can't manage, or get through life without constantly suppressing unresolved trauma despite the signals in your mental and physical health.

Harmful coping habits creep in and make our situation feel even more out of control. The hamful habits I hear of in my clinical practice are of eating too much of the wrong foods, substance abuse from alcohol or other drugs, and generally people not taking care of themselves.

Being stuck in a downward coping spiral accumulates with a range of unwanted side effects like digestive pain, brain fog, poor sleep, low energy, anxiety and weight gain. It can be so frustrating when you *do* take steps towards positive changes, they don't work for long.

The reason these steps don't work long-term is that there is no "one-size-fits-all" health approach for the lifestyles of this complicated modern world. Your strategy will not work unless your time and effort are personalised to the unique needs of your mind and body.

Getting out of this survival mode starts with knowing what's going on, so you can do something about it. There are many factors at play here, which we will explore in this book, but the over-arching issue for those of us who live with chronic stress or unresolved trauma is we have a dysregulated nervous system, which means we are stuck in a "fight and flight" mode, even when there's no current threat.

Your central nervous system (CNS) is made up of the brain and spinal cord, governed as part of your autonomic nervous system. This is your main control centre to detect safety or threats. It lets you know when you can feel at ease and function healthily, and when you need to be on alert.

The branch of the CNS that lets you know when to be on alert is the sympathetic nervous system, known as the "fight and flight" mode. This state is most activated when your brain senses a threat. It's the survival mode that mobilises you to take action by increasing your heart rate and blood flow to your muscles. Think of when you're driving in the car and someone in front of you slams their brakes on to avoid someone else on the road. We need this system to protect us and others from harm, but it's exhausting to be in "fight and flight" mode all the time. Our nervous system needs to reset to the parasympathetic mode – also known as "rest and digest" – after this kind of hyperalert experience to give us balance and ease. Think of this state as the parachute that's meant to slow you down and ground you. This state replenishes your energy and allows for healing and repair.

If you've been dealing with overwhelming stress or unresolved trauma, your brain can learn to overprotect you. It can become normalised or sensitised to this survival stress mode even when the threat is gone. Similar to when a car alarm goes off even when no one is near it, your dysregulated nervous system is throwing out "threat" responses to neutral inputs from around or within you.

How and why we respond in the way we do is largely due to our bio-individuality. This includes our current health status, unique personality traits, previously unresolved traumas, social support and genetic makeup (DNA).

If we live with unresolved trauma, we need to recognise and acknowledge the emotions that experiences evoke in us. It takes time to process and understand how it has affected us in our social connections too. Carrying pain from unresolved post-traumatic stress can be a major barrier to building meaningful connections. In my practice, I hear from people all the time that it's hard to trust others, including sources of information that might help us to get unstuck.

Many people I've worked with over the years don't easily filter overstimulation or demands of our modern world. If you're like them you might relate to being highly sensitive to the emotions of others and environmental substances, including foods, noise or smells. These sensitivities tend to be common in those who have personality traits of highly sensitive people, or empaths. If you are aware of the effects of these genetic personality traits and their unique nervous system needs, you can strengthen this gift, reset faster and prevent many physical challenges that can occur if ignored. I'll describe why and how to strengthen the traits of a highly sensitive person in Chapter 3.

Foundations of Repair and Recovery

Let's use one example of an approach to restoring a damaged house after a storm. You wouldn't start with the roof if you didn't even have the walls up. You want to start with establishing solid foundations to make the restoration last. If you have a blueprint or house plans, it's like having a map to follow for the best results. Similarly, your greatest ability to influence your health starts with knowing how to support the foundations found in the genetic imprint of your DNA. When you live in a way that is aligned to support your DNA you can take steps forward in the right order to improve your resilience.

DNA is often referred to as the molecule of life and is found in almost all of your cells. DNA is the instruction manual that helps build and run our bodies. Our genes are sections of DNA (deoxyribonucleic acid) that have a chemical code, to make specific proteins.

These proteins make different cells that make us look, think and feel like our unique selves. Our DNA is what makes us all human – yet different from each other.

This DNA code is like a set of instructions that influences how different parts of our body grow, develop and function which then impacts how we handle traumatic events. Other environmental factors can also play a role in how well we recover from those experiences. If our health is not aligned with the needs of our DNA it can make it more difficult to bounce back from difficult situations.

The new science of epigenetics is teaching us that our genes can be healthy or sick, just like we can. Our genes are exquisitely sensitive to how we treat them. They are guided in part by the foods we eat, how we think and our choice of lifestyle.

Since 2012, my clinical work has revolved around problem-solving complex health cases, specialising in natural treatments for disorders in gut–brain interaction. A wish to explore new methods for faster results led me to train in the interpretation of DNA test profiles. Emerging research and widespread test availability highlighted primary pathways of clinically important genes that can influence our quality of health.

Insights from hundreds of DNA testing cases helped me see patterns of dysfunction that were related to the same body systems over and over again. Nine genes consistently held the most influence when it came to helping my patients create new behaviours through better gut and brain function. These nine genes are what I delve into in this book.

Gaining insights from these genes and strengthening your gut–brain function will help unlock your DNA potential, reset your nervous system and restore your health. It's like a framework for you to prioritise your actions in daily food choices and lifestyle activities to support your health. This strategy is more motivating, enjoyable and sustainable than a one-size-fits-all solution. By focusing on practical awareness, making intentional choices about food and lifestyle, and cultivating a sense of safety and trust, we can recreate healthy patterns and find lasting healing. Let me guide you in the right direction.

I am not the only one to suggest that the ways we eat, think and live affects our DNA function and health outcomes. I am building on decades of research. Without these other researchers and their pioneering work, hundreds of positive results in my clinical work wouldn't have happened.

This book brings pieces of the puzzle together to offer solutions to help align your unique biological needs to a lifestyle that supports healing from adversity. I've developed and refined a framework called C.A.R.E., which has helped numerous people I've worked with, who were stuck in many areas of their health and life – until they had new insights and a reason to apply this strategy to *their* genes and situation. Some of their stories are in this book. *Their names and identifying details have been changed to protect the privacy of individuals.*

What Kind of Clinician Am I?

I am a naturopath and clinical nutritionist. Naturopathy is a science-based system that uses natural interventions to support healing the body and mind. Similar to functional medicine, its aim is address the underlying causes of imbalance rather than treat just treat the symptoms. This means the focus is on a personalised eating plan that addresses short and long term goals. Natural methods to support healing may include herbal medicines or supplements and lifestyle strategies to support sleep, detoxification and stress management.

HOW TO USE THIS BOOK

This book is divided into three sections that build on one another.

Part One – Identify
Explains the relationship with your mind–body signals, unique genetic personality traits and how these affect the way your nervous system responds during stress.

Part Two – Interpret
Looks at the foundational causes to approach if there is an imbalance in any of three key areas, represented as a three-legged stool:

1. Quality of digestion impacting cells
2. Specific needs of brain (physiology)
3. Genetic risk for addictive behaviours.

You will learn the connection imbalances in any of these areas may have with your current signals, and the corresponding genes to prioritise for support.

Part Three – Implement
Lifestyle principles and dietary actions to restore your long-term health, based on the totality of nine gene traits discussed in this book.

You can read this book cover to cover or dip in and out of parts that interest you. If you read from cover to cover, you might notice some points repeated from different angles. The chapters are designed this way for non-linear readers who prefer to dip into different chapters of the book.

You may be tempted to start with the lifestyle, food changes or recipes right away, although knowing *why* it's beneficial to live this way makes this process more motivating and sustainable. When you identify with your possible gene variations and behavioural patterns, this connection can help you make and adjust food and activity choices to the current needs of your mind or body.

You'll find suggested activities, support groups and assessments to explore in the resources list at the end.

Note: For ease of reading and fewer distractions, I've listed the research in notes at the end of the book, rather than within the text.

PART ONE — IDENTIFY

To get unstuck we need to *identify the real problem* behind painful signals calling our attention through challenging emotions, behaviours or bodily sensations. Those unresolved thoughts and feelings can have a residual cost on our health and relationships. When we acknowledge them as a message of need, we can curiously start *to dig deeper*.

This section will introduce you to a map for identifying the factors that contribute to overwhelm:

1. Allostatic load – the cumulative stress of too much pressure
2. Epigenetics – the combined impact of our genes and current lifestyle
3. Perspective – how we frame our thinking and stories

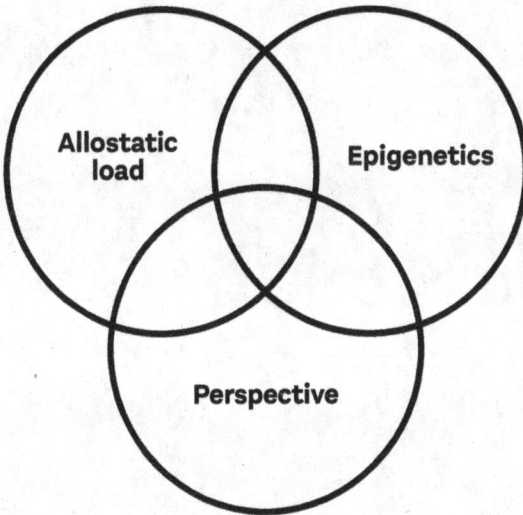

p`phcal injuy but emotional psychological ... "... of"`

— 1 —
MEANINGFUL
SIGNALS

*"The body is the container
of all our sensations and feelings"*
—Dr. Peter Levine

Nervous System Signalling

Every human brain, by design, has an inbuilt survival need to detect danger at all times. It's part of the primitive, protective wiring of our nervous system that's kept us alive throughout human history. When threatened, this natural human response creates an imprint in the cellular memory of our body. Many leading trauma experts say a person's body needs to later resolve these imprints to fully heal. You'll find some of these experts in the resources section at the end of this book.

All of us, in different ways, experience some type of trauma throughout life. Maybe you wouldn't use the term "trauma" to describe your past circumstances. I know I didn't for many years. The real essence of trauma, though, originates with the same Greek word meaning a "wound or hurt". It doesn't relate to only physical injury but emotional too. It can affect the body, mind, or spirit, or all at once. We can't visually see an injury to our mind or spirit the same as we can see a cut or a bruise. This is what makes emotional trauma difficult to quantify.

According to trauma expert Dr. Gabor Mate in his book *When the Body Says No*, "trauma is not just what happened to us, it's more about the impact within us related to what happened or neglected to happen to us."

All emotions, either expressed or not, always affect our physical health. Our emotional wounds need attention to heal just the same. Especially, when all life experiences involve some degree of emotional response.

My former mentor used to say, "Our issues are stored in our tissues." In other words, our memories or issues from past physical or emotional traumas remain stored in us, in our biology. Unless they are released or resolved through our nervous system, our body remembers.

The impact of unresolved trauma goes deeper. Often affecting our ability to trust our innate wisdom. This relates to what psychiatrist Dr. Bessel A van der Kolk, describes in his book *The Body Keeps the Score,* as how traumatised people often feel unsafe in their bodies. This constant internal discomfort from the past teaches many to become numb and ignore their gut feelings.

I certainly experienced this. I lost some trust in my own inner guidance after my China incident in 2008 and this led me to lose confidence in knowing who I could rely on. As a result, I became less social, resourceful and willing to seek help. The surest thing I could trust was spending time in nature. Nature, to me, is always a place to find inspiration and a reminder of the divine.

When we return to our usual day-to-day life we can be reminded of those past hurts, through heavy emotions or physical pains that seemingly appear out of the blue. For many, suppressing uncomfortable signals works for a while, however, the way we behave at home or relate to others usually changes.

In my clinical work, as I learnt approaches to help others improve their health problems, countless times there were clear patterns of unresolved emotional trauma. Unintentionally, this was how I realised a connection between my own behaviours and unresolved traumatic stress. Once we recognise the connection it's hard to ignore.

What should be done? Where should I start?

Before trying to solve the problems that come up in life, identify the real issues. It's easy to focus on symptoms and not causes. We need to investigate more deeply, under the surface.

We can look at health symptoms with the analogy of a train journey.

Symptoms act as a predictor of the train track – showing where we're heading. Our body and mind leave clues or signals in the form of clinical patterns or diagnoses. These patterns once connected, tell us how we got on this train. This is especially useful for symptoms like brain fog, digestive pain, fatigue, muscle spasms, anxiety, depression, poor sleep, weight problems and more. These are all early warning signals to investigate, for there are underlying causes.

With the right strategy, it's possible to slow down the train we're on. By implementing a new lifestyle with sustainable actions it's more likely we can even switch onto a completely different train track. With that picture in mind, let's investigate more deeply.

Finding Misalignment

If you don't release difficult emotions, a state of dis-ease can surface in your physical body. Your symptoms are a message, a call for help from your mind and body. There's meaning behind them and, when you identify that, the insight can give you the ability to ask better questions rather than ignore the message.

For thousands of years in traditional Eastern medicine, both Chinese and Ayurvedic, specific organs are understood to correspond with certain emotions. Think of the saying, "The weight of the world is on someone's shoulders." Pain in this area, and also the neck, concerns our responsibilities. The lower back and spine are about how supported we feel or how we support ourselves. The liver relates to anger, resentment, shame or frustration. The lungs are connected to the emotion of grief. Our stomach and belly, being our centre of personal power, usually connect to the deep emotional expression of unspoken feelings. The breasts are self-nurturing, and the ovaries and uterus are linked with creativity. Our knees allow us to step forward and are connected to the fear of movement or aging.

Psychotherapist and author of the book, *Emotional Sensitivity*, Imi Lo says, "The old health paradigm is linear and says that symptoms are bad and need to be eradicated. The new paradigm says that the discomforts are signals from our deepest self, that it is time to change. Teaching us something. "

Symptoms appear as feedback in different forms, such as phys-ical, mental or emotional discomfort or tension. Feelings like fear or anxiety are types of signals. Signals are a way to communicate in any language. Like any language, when we understand it, then we can interpret it as important or minor.

Research on the autonomic nervous system calls this ability

to interpret our symptoms, interoception. It is the sensing and understanding of internal signals coming from our body. Think of it simply as our subconscious asking the question "How do I feel?" from moment to moment. The better we're able to listen to and distinguish between different sensations, signals or emotions, the more accurately we'll know how to handle them. The easiest ones to tune into are the physical signals of hunger or thirst.

Here's an example of a typical pattern for a busy person I often see in my clinic, let's call her Grace. Some days Grace is so focused on the tasks at hand, various meetings, driving kids around or caring for others that she can run through the day and forget to eat! While getting everything done, she might feel those first signs of hunger but she'll steamroll over them because something else needs her attention. By the time she gets home, she's not only physically hungry but mentally exhausted. It's easy to resort to something to "soothe" her. Once she's finally able to relax, Grace binges on anything in front of her that doesn't need any effort to cook. Things like quick processed carbs: toast, cookies and cereals. She then overeats before going to bed which disturbs her sleep and sets her up for less energy to choose nourishing foods the next day.

It's easy to see how we learn to ignore our internal physical and emotional signals. We can become overwhelmed with the distractions of modern life, when we're conditioned to be productive, to do more and keep up.

More intense painful signals are harder to ignore. At some point, you might not be able to push through or avoid what your body is calling attention to. With some deeper, quiet reflection there may be something else not aligned between the needs of the inner (mind–body) and outer (external) world. What else might be missing? Perhaps other needs are lacking balance? Is there a lack of quiet time alone to do the things that make you happy, like taking a relaxing bath or making your favourite meal? For those who already have too much alone time perhaps the right social connections are needed to fill an emotional gap. It will be different for each of us at different times. One thing is for sure with either situation, caring for your wellbeing has to come from a place of kindness and not punishment. It is about regularly taking action to nurture your health and happiness. Implementing some of the lifestyle activities and food choices you will learn in Part 3 are positive actions to support any core deficiencies even if you can't identify them yet.

In our modern world, which is so focused on the physical body, the usual approach is often a numbers game. Track your weight, calories, steps, and heart rate to see if you're "normal". So many of us have forgotten what it is like to feel healthy and happy. Most people, unless their parents are health professionals, haven't learned how to interpret the early signals of discomfort in our minds or bodies. If we have a headache, we are told, "to take a painkiller and make it go away." With more serious aches and pains that do not go away by suppressing them alone, we often normalise them as part of life. Many people unknowingly accept a pretty low standard of feeling well. However, this does not have to be a fixed state forever. Misinterpreting your body's signals in the past is certainly not your fault!

Mainstream education today generally doesn't teach classes on body awareness, traditional healing principles or even the latest nutrition research. These are all learnable skills though. When we prioritise actions after identifying underlying deficiencies, it builds momentum to keep on improving. This generates hope for a new reality. If we practice slowing down, being present more often and emotionally tuning in to what's triggering us, we have a chance to empower ourselves.

Ancient Japanese wisdom reveals a beautiful metaphor for healing and recovery from adversity. *Kintsugi* is a legend believed to date back to the 15th Century. This Japanese artistic practice, which translates literally as "golden joinery", involves putting broken pottery pieces back together with gold. The legend came about when a mighty shogun warrior broke his favourite tea bowl and sent it off for repairs. The first repair was disappointing to the shogun. After a new craftsman added gold to the cracks, the warrior thought it added to the bowl's value and beauty.

It's a wonderful reminder to embrace our imperfections, teaching us that those parts make us more beautiful, and once repaired, we can be stronger because of the breaks. Author of *Kintsugi Wellness*, Candice Kumai says, "The struggles will become your story, and that's the beauty of *kintsugi*. Your cracks can become the most beautiful part of you."

The Overwhelm Map

During those intensely difficult times that we all experience, it may seem, at least on the outside, that we have got it all together. Beneath the surface, is another picture. Overwhelm peaks when you can no longer ignore the uncomfortable attention those signals are making.

A collision of three main factors sets the stage. What I call the overwhelm map. Similar to other maps, there are different routes to get to your destination. You have some influence over all of them and can choose which factor to focus on first. If you know how you got to where you are, then you've got a reference point for where to pay more attention, so you have a way to get out.

1. Allostatic load – the cumulative stress of too much pressure
2. Epigenetics – the combined impact of our genes and current lifestyle
3. Perspective – how we frame our thinking and stories

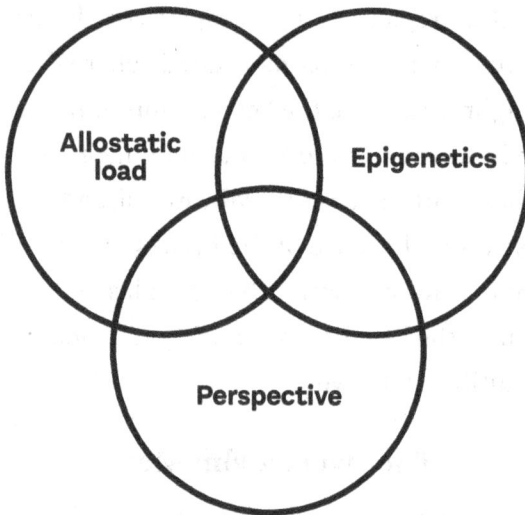

Let's take a look at each of these.

1. Allostatic Load – why can't we handle the pressure
Our health risks are influenced by our own accumulated stressful life experiences and those inherited from our ancestors – in our genes. Our genes then affect our ability to handle stress and adapt to change. Without interventions, our cells' energy capacity and

demand can be impacted in ways that make us more susceptible to feeling overwhelmed or stuck in the long term. The stress response can be set off by various sources, including physical injury, infection or emotional trauma – both real and perceived threats.

Endocrinologist Hans Selye discovered this in 1936, believing that when faced with excessive stress the gut, along with the endocrine and immune systems, become altered in response to chemical and physical challenges. Selye's theory emphasises the importance of balance and highlights that excessive stress occurs when "demands placed on an organism exceed its reasonable capacity to fulfil them".

This stress theory was further developed as the allostatic load by Sterling and Eyer in 1981. This concept refers to our ability to maintain stability through change.

When we reach a point where we can't maintain that stability anymore all our hormones and inflammatory systems are impacted, which can present issues such as brain fog, weight struggles, poor sleep and mood swings.

2. Epigenetics – how lifestyle affects our genes

The second factor in the overwhelm map is how we respond based on our genes and lifestyle.

Recent advances in genetic technology and research have allowed us to uncover much more than where our ancestors came from or defects related to medical genetics. Scientists now understand that our genes influence our physical and psychological strengths as well as our risk for certain health issues.

The importance of your influence of control on your genetic code starts with understanding how DNA connects with our cells, which makes us who we are. Your DNA (genetic code) gives instructions to your cells, telling them what to do based on their environment. Think of it as the user's manual for a car.

Cells are the foundation for all living things.

Inside almost every cell of our body is a chemical substance called deoxyribonucleic acid (DNA).

Each gene is a short section of DNA.

Our DNA makes different proteins that make our cells work in unique ways that shape who we are.

Our human genome is made up of 20,000–25,000 genes, which control our development from a single cell into a complex, adult body.

There are only slight differences in our human DNA code but enough that make us each unique. None of us have the exact same DNA unless we're identical twins. Yet when it comes to food, sleep and lifestyle habits we're all given the same 'one size fits all' message.

Our gene code structure remains fixed for life. Although our power to make changes that influence the way our genes act or function is flexible. This is where epigenetics comes in. Researchers in this field of study now understand that all outside influences including diet, environmental inputs, lifestyle habits, family history and all past personal experiences affect the functioning of our genes. Think of it as the accumulated effect of everything you put into your body, how you move, rest and socially connect. These inputs, technically called epigenomes, change the way our DNA instructions are read by different cells and have been shown to pass from one generation to the next without any change in the genes themselves.

Information in our DNA is stored as a code made up of four chemical bases: adenine (A), guanine (G), cytosine (C) and thymine

(T), labelled as A, C, G, and T for ease. Each gene code makes an enzyme (a protein). Variations in the position of just one of these bases in a DNA chain could make a difference in the function of that enzyme and how your body works. This variation in the gene code is called a single nucleotide polymorphism (SNP) and basically is like a spelling change in a word. Similar to how the meaning of a word changes if we write C-A-T verses C-A-G. Having gene variants in our DNA code is normal and no human is without them.

Gene variants affect the speed a gene functions at and pathways of related body systems. These variants are not called "defects" or mutations as in medical genetics.

Understanding which genes need more help and how gives insights into making better choices to help them function well. Think of how a sports coach might set up a team to play a game. A better game strategy might be to focus on supporting the weakest players on the team to improve rather than strengthening the players who are already doing well. It's a simple analogy that helps us bring a holistic view to health and how our human body performs or responds to life.

Genes have a hierarchy; they are not all equal in their influence. Some gene pathways affect several hundred genes while others very few. Certain groups of genes code for our response to inflammation, fat metabolism, mental health and many more.

Our genes influence every behavioural trait we have. Research shows we even inherit temperaments. Whether we have any musical ear ability or not, and if we have any predisposed health risks alongside potential gifts, are in our genetic instruction code. When bundled together, several groups of genetic traits shape our personality. Personality is described as a person's set of characteristics that are relatively consistent across situations. Making the connection that our genes influence our personality means you have some control over who your future self can be.

3. Perspective – how we frame our thinking and stories

It's often hard to see another perspective when we experience painful or traumatic events. With time, reflecting on a different viewpoint is crucial though. The way we view our experiences and mindset has a profound effect on our physical and mental health.

Our power to change things for the better is largely found in our thinking patterns or stories we tell ourselves and others – whether we're aware of it or not. The good news is that we can reframe our stories if we are open and willing to view things differently.

When we understand our role, we gain some control. Our role each day starts with the quality of our thoughts and then follows with actions. If left unaware or unconscious of the role of our mindset, we may stay stuck longer.

Think of a different viewpoint similar to putting on different eyeglasses. The new lenses can alter the story we tell ourselves. A supportive team of qualified therapists, such as psychotherapists, counsellors and psychologists, can accelerate the process.

The Key to Change

Understanding your own overwhelm map is the key to change. Rather than focusing on symptoms, you will be able to address three factors that work behind the scenes to create those symptoms: Your stress load with your current state of health, a combination of your genes and lifestyle, and your personal perspective of your situation. Gaining insights into these is the first step in regaining control of your health. But the next piece we need to understand is what your baseline of mind-body health really is, and how this impacts on your stress load.

— 2 —
UNDERSTANDING "NORMAL" IS NOT NATURAL

"There comes a point where we need to stop just pulling people out of the river. We need to go upstream and find out why they're falling in."
— Desmond Tutu

What is Old is New

Awareness of the mind–body connection is by no means new. Until approximately 300 years ago, virtually every system of medicine throughout the world treated the mind, body and emotions as an interrelated whole. All classic medical texts, from the Daoist classics of traditional Chinese medicine to Ayurvedic texts to writings from Hippocrates, have encouraged us to regard food as a vital part of medicine. Up until 150 years ago, pharmaceutical drugs did not exist.

It was during the 17th Century that the Western world started to see mind and body as two distinct entities. In this view, the body was seen as a machine, complete with replaceable, independent parts, with no connection whatsoever to the mind. This Western viewpoint had definite benefits, acting as the foundation for advances in surgery, trauma care, pharmaceuticals, and other areas of allopathic medicine. However, it also greatly reduced scientific inquiry into humans' emotional and spiritual life and downplayed our innate ability to heal.

In more recent years this view gradually started to return to appreciating ancient wisdom. Research into mind–body connections is now validating what existed for thousands of years, and demonstrating the complex links between the body and mind.

Ayurveda is an ancient healing system of India with the central philosophy that physical health cannot be achieved without emotional, mental and spiritual health. Traditional Chinese medicine regards balancing four pillars of diet, movement, adequate rest and good mental attitude (which encompasses mind and spirit) as the foundations of health.

If you're wondering why you haven't heard a more empowering message about looking after your health, you're not alone. What and where we listen to our information is largely dependent on our environment. Who are you listening to? Is it mainstream TV, radio news, or a well-intended suggestion from a friend or family member? Are you able to listen to other opinions but filter out any that don't align with your values?

I had a first-hand insight into what influences mainstream health messages while studying at the Brain Institute at the University of Queensland in 2015. After graduating with all distinctions in my health science degree in 2010 I initially felt my calling was in research. I was lucky to be accepted among only a dozen others into an advanced neuroscience degree. It sounded ideal to have extra credibility to my passion for nutrition research on improving brain function through having this experience at the Brain Institute. Back then, widespread recognition was emerging that our brain function wasn't fixed, as once believed in the past. Neuroplasticity was a newly accepted term and this fascinated me. My grandmother lost her life to a neurodegenerative brain disease with few treatment options available at the time, so it was a very personal motivation.

A couple of months into the Master's degree I excitedly compiled a handful of recent research papers I'd accessed on key nutrients and meditation for improving brain health. My professor pondered them for a few days and came back to me with an unexpected response. He said it was interesting to know but the course's grant funding was for developing pharmaceutical drugs for treating dementia. He said I'd need to wait until finishing a PhD before digging into the research field I was most interested in.

I left feeling disheartened and realised I couldn't wait that long – my voice would be silenced and I'd have to put years of effort into study that didn't align with my heart or values for helping others. I know from courses I have studied on ancient health systems like Ayurveda and traditional Chinese medicine, that the principles of safely using the best of nature should be an empowering choice we hear more often.

This experience confirmed what I'd suspected and heard about "big money" investments coming from large industries, like pharmaceuticals. This funding drives messages we hear from our governments via the media, and flows to the education passed onto our medical teams. Shortly after that conversation with my professor I withdrew from the University of Queensland and started my own business in clinical practice.

I remembered I'd had a glimpse into a totally different health approach used only about 100 years ago. On a guided walking tour in my travels to Singapore, I was taken to an old Chinatown area where early Chinese settlers lived around the 1920s. It was fascinating to discover doctors using Chinese medicine were paid a retainer to keep patients healthy. If a patient became sick, the doctor would not be paid until the patient's health returned. An important notion of traditional Chinese medicine was disease prevention and maintaining health. The ancient Chinese believed it was "devilish" and inhumane to take fees from a sick person who was very limited in what they could do because they were sick. Thus the major function of traditional Chinese doctors, the same as in naturopathic medicine, is that of a teacher and educator.

Non-communicable diseases account for about 70% of all deaths globally. These come from the main conditions of chronic disease: Cardiovascular diseases, cancers, chronic obstructive pulmonary disease (COPD) and diabetes. Our modifiable behaviours like an unhealthy diet, smoking, physical inactivity and harmful alcohol use all increase our risk of chronic disease. Identifying the behaviours you can influence is a crucial key. You have some control over your choices when you learn the knowledge of ways to reduce your risk of chronic disease. While it may be idealistic to consider our modern health system to adopt something similar to ancient Chinese, where the doctor is paid when you are well and not when you are sick, we would likely see a re-emergence of our personal responsibility to wellness become a higher priority.

What Does True Health Look And Feel Like?

The people I see in my practice are those who want to take charge of their health and prevent a worsening quality of life. They usually pay attention to early signals or are fed up with results from using other methods. They won't accept a health diagnosis if they think or intuitively feel that it is not the only solution best for them.

I work in the wellness and empowerment space, so all too often I hear others comment, "My doctor says my blood results are all fine (normal), but I don't feel good. I don't feel like myself anymore."

When I met Marie, she was one of them too, yet described herself as "not really having any symptoms." She just wanted to know how to feel her best again. Except, upon more questioning, it turned out she had itchy skin sometimes, regular gas and bloating and PMS. In reality, she was experiencing a lot more discomfort than she was initially willing to acknowledge. Her body was sending signals that something wasn't right, although she thought it was "normal female stuff." Her sister had similar experiences, so it was seen as a family thing.

Many uncomfortable states of health are accepted as normal or just part of the ageing process in today's Western world. Quite different views on health and ageing exist in some African and Eastern cultures, where the wise village elder is a central part of the community.

Especially common for modern women are the symptoms of hormone imbalance, which greatly reduces their quality of life. In 2022, the largest study to date on the day-to-day health and metabolism of menopausal women found that 82% of more than 6000 women reported poor sleep as their most common symptom. Other common symptoms of hormone imbalances are mood swings and dips in energy. Statistics on recent surveys and research studies indicate at least 50% of Western women aged 35–60 (perimenopause and postmenopausal) have a combination of symptoms.

With our aging population, the North American Menopause

Society estimates that worldwide 1.1 billion women will be in the transition to menopause or post-menopausal by the year 2025. Identifying causes of hormone balance and interventions to improve symptoms will benefit many now and in the future.

It's difficult to grasp that normal isn't the same as natural (in a historical sense). The norm just refers to what is common nowadays and what many people are experiencing. Think about how we use or accept that word – normal doesn't mean it's supposed to be there. These symptoms are signals from our body that something isn't right. Some people say, 'Oh, it's just part of being a female.'

Is it though?

Maybe it's part of being a modern woman but it wasn't before and doesn't have to be.

This extreme change has escalated in the last 50 years or so through a combination of several dietary and lifestyle factors that shifted many of us, in urban living in Western countries, towards an inflammatory health bias. In that time, some important things to advance us towards "better living" have been introduced into our everyday environment. Compared to previous generations, we're now living in a more toxic environment. Synthetic chemicals are being put in our gardens and parks, our food (both fresh and processed), cosmetics, and cleaning products are being fed to the animals and fish that we eat. We spend hours in front of digital screens and live in concrete urban settings with heavy traffic, pollution and neon lights keeping us awake until all hours of the night. Our immune system, which mostly resides in our gut (digestive tract), treats all of these chemicals as invaders and inflames our whole system.

Social dynamics shifted with women moving into the workplace while retaining all other responsibilities. It's no wonder the typical answer for keeping up with this pace is using pain-relieving medication or pushing through the poor sleep or other overwhelming issues most of us feel. Or temporarily escape the pain with an excess of unhealthy food or drink to help lift our mood. Most of these contemporary ailments are accepted as normal. Though as I indicated earlier, what's normal isn't necessarily natural.

What is natural is when the body and the mind function well together. Symptoms have become more common, as our society has shifted away from what is natural. So, reconnecting with nature's rhythms along with connecting with our inner nature is the starting point. What this means practically is realigning oneself with simple day-to-day habits to feel like part of nature. We need to understand the body's natural design. Working with the design means we don't have to be slaves to the symptoms. With the right awareness and actions, it's possible to feel consistently well most of the time. Life doesn't have to always feel crazy and out of balance.

We are all part of nature *and* made of the same particles as the ocean, trees, mountains, animals and stars. We are not separate from it. All of nature works in a cycle – the sun rises and sets, seasons come and go, the moon cycles every month, and planets shift. Our digestion has a cycle. Our sleep works in a cycle. Feeling symptom-free depends on how closely each of us aligns with nature's rhythms.

To increase internal awareness it is good to ask ourselves, "What do I do that disconnects me from nature?" From time to time, I can also relate to some of the usual suspects like excessive use of electronics, imbalanced or irregular eating, eating in front of the TV, eating processed foods, irregular sleep patterns, not spending time daily in nature, or having enough time in natural light. These are all the things we do that get in the way of our bodies connecting with nature's patterns. This combination is the perfect storm to contribute to all the symptoms I often see in hormone and energy imbalances – easy weight gain, poor sleep, and more.

Everything we do matters. Everything we eat, think and do today affects our mind and body in the future. Our entire physical body is always in a state of transition. Shedding the old and creating the new.

Clues to Identify Gaps

It's fair to say that if you don't feel right or have ongoing symptoms, this is an internal clue you must trust and investigate before accepting the first opinion you received on standard bloodwork. Answers you receive can differ widely depending on the field and focus of training your health professional uses.

As adults, we're told it's best to get an annual check-up with our doctor. Typically, I'll see people after their doctors have run some basic blood panels and are told that everything is fine. Many people don't understand what these blood tests actually measure. Metabolic markers for hormones that impact weight and risk for diabetes are often not requested as part of a medical check-up or patients are not given the actual numbers or test results.

When it comes to identifying if your lab results are indeed optimal, it's best to look beyond the line of "fine."

The reference ranges used in pathology are determined based on the average health of a local population at that time. So, if the majority of the population in your country is currently metabolically unhealthy, that is the standard. That means what's "normal" or "fine" is far from optimal. If your results show you are on the borderline of a reference range, then likely some metabolic dysfunction is *already* going on.

Studies also show that people with a family history of psychological problems or who have been through significant stress recently tend to, on average, have nutrient levels lower than those without that problem, but lab testing would still show them as being within the "normal range." So the term "deficiency" in nutrients should be personalised. You might have a nutrient deficiency relative to your own metabolic needs rather than being deficient compared to the general population. In other words, you can be within the normal range for the general population, but not the normal range for you individually, meaning you may not be getting enough for your body and brain.

Ideal Range Biomarkers

For you to feel empowered with your health it's crucial to know where you're at in your metabolic health.

This gives you a starting point to track your data and to stay motivated by the progress of any changes you make. Metabolic health is foundational as it affects everything from energy to mental focus, mood, weight control and sleep quality. If you know the optimal reference ranges for some key biomarkers, it can bring the pieces of your health puzzle together faster to detect early decline and improve your daily quality of health.

Optimal health references are different from pathology ranges. A classic example of range variation that's especially important is fasting insulin. This is a key biomarker for metabolic function and insulin resistance that is not always requested in routine bloodwork.

The ideal or optimal range is <5 but the acceptable pathology range is <15.

Another easy home alternative to check for insulin resistance is the waist-to-height ratio measurement, using a tape measure. Research indicates that a healthy waist-to-height ratio ranges between 0.4 to 0.49.

A ratio of 0.5 to 0.59 puts people at increased risk of metabolic health problems, while a waist-to-height ratio of 0.6 or more places people at the highest risk of disease.

As an example, a woman who is 1.65 meters tall with a waist circumference of 76 cm will be 76 ÷ 165 = 0.46, and considered relatively healthy. However if her waist above 83 cm that will put her into the unhealthy range.

Here's how easy it is to measure your waist measurement:
- Find the midpoint between the bottom of your ribs and the top of your hips. Just above your navel.
- Wrap the tape measure closely against your skin.
- Breathe out naturally and take your measurement.
- Repeat one more time for accuracy.

Realistically you want to know at what health stage you're in to have an idea of when to expect successful lasting results when you try new lifestyle treatment methods. The three stages of health care are:
1. Symptomatic (gets you feeling better – mild relief)
2. Corrective Care (explores underlying causes)
3. Wellness Care (prevention and maintenance to stay well)

The Right Time and Place
for the Modern Medical System

Modern medical health care still plays an important role. I'm not suggesting we should be without it. Where would we be without the many fast-acting benefits of modern medicine? Western medicinal methods can be incredible for keeping our vital signs alive. Like when acute conditions arise from infections, toxins, cardiac arrest and many other emergencies that require urgent attention from accidents such as blood loss, cuts or broken bones. In these situations, hospitals and a Western medical approach are incredible.

In the right moments having access to surgery, anaesthetics, early detection screening through medical technology, obstetrics and trauma care (including some medications to keep you alive) is extremely useful. Specialists with skills in these fields are the best for survival and rehabilitation after crisis care. Over 200 years of medical advancements have resulted in some of these incredible methods being widely available. It's akin to giving someone a life jacket when they're drowning. Useful short term, but getting them out of the water and back on safe land to walk again (teaching them how to stay healthy), is better in the long term.

The people who come to see me are those who take action to fix the quality of their health that affects their daily lives because it is of high value to them. Many of these people have seen that when it comes to chronic diseases, especially mental health states (like anxiety or depression), digestive imbalances, diabetes, and many other hormone or autoimmune diseases, our Western health system isn't set up to treat the real cause.

For conditions that affect our quality of life, the results aren't there. It's not a comment I say without substance. Education for nutrition, food, or mind–body awareness isn't the basis of our standard healthcare system today. As endocrinologist Dr. Robert Lustig states so well in his book *Metabolical*, "we can't treat a food problem with a drug." What's been done to our foods, through processing and growing chemicals affects everything to do with our health.

Almost all traditional and Eastern healing systems emphasise individualised nutrition from real food choices and alongside lifestyle behaviours. Yet nutrition isn't taught in most medical schools across the world. Modern medicine specialists and doctors are taught – this is the diagnosis (pathophysiology), treatment and pills (medications). Unless you fit into a category within the disease state, you'll be dismissed or perhaps given antidepressants to help your sleep or mood. In fairness to the modern general practitioner, the system isn't set up to give them time to ask questions about what you eat, regular physical activity, how much sleep you get, or any emotional stress.

Our buying habits in the supermarket aren't questioned or factored in. We live in a food environment today that is very harmful to health with sugary drinks, and highly palatable packaged products that can sit on the shelf for months or years and are still called food. Many people falsely believe it's cheaper to eat that way, but everything in life eventually has a payoff.

The long-term costs in time spent being active with friends or family, lost opportunities at work or even our peace of mind are real when quality of health declines. While today's mainstream healthcare is more like a disease-management system that lacks patient empowerment and transference of education, improvements are surfacing. The growing popularity of functional medicine in the past decade indicates our mainstream healthcare may once again provide holistic and personalised treatment approaches that acknowledge the importance of our mind and body messages – key elements of Eastern traditional medicines.

The Power of Better Questions

We all need help at certain times in our lives. At each stage the need for new support, different tools or better options becomes obvious. The difficulty of living with ongoing pain (physical, mental or emotional) can become unbearable if we don't explore other options. I invite you to explore. Experience and experiment with safe, time-tested methods that support the mind–body connection and bridge the gap between historical views and modern science.

Moving away from what's normal but not natural takes some reflection and courage. By asking more specific questions of your health provider it puts you in the driving seat with what's really going on when you don't feel "fine", as is often said when reviewing bloodwork.

Then start with questioning ingredients used or food sources at the places you eat or in food products you buy. Awareness of food quality versus quantity can be an eye-opening skill.

As you progress you may start to question how you feel. Spend a few minutes each day, checking in to notice any changes in sensations related to either energy or pain that might be related to what you ate or avoided.

Connecting the dots isn't usually an easy journey. Anything truly transformational rarely is. Lasting relief and empowering results can be yours if you're willing to try and explore.

Next, we will bring together the other piece of the puzzle that's possibly contributing to your situation of being overwhelmed – inherited personality traits. Our traits come with both gifts and challenges.

— 3 —
SUPPRESSED SENSITIVITY TRAITS

"Knowing yourself is the beginning of all wisdom"
— Aristotle

What's on the Inside Matters Most

I work with many high-achieving professional women in my clinic, "superwomen", who pride themselves on willpower, discipline and results in many areas of their lives. They come to me with symptoms such as poor sleep, mood swings, brain fog or weight struggles, which they can't get on top of no matter how hard they try. These outwardly strong, warrior-type women are usually very emotionally sensitive. Many have toughened up to succeed in a work role or fit in with the norms of society. Suppressing our feminine side and sensitivity for a long time can sabotage health and sometimes relationships.

We live in a world that pushes the "see before we believe" message. Unless we can smell, touch, see, hear or taste something, it doesn't exist. Recognition by at least one of the five sensory systems makes it "real" and there's barely any acknowledgment of our innate sixth sense. Yet all humans are born with an intuitive connection to everything and everyone around us.

Maybe you can remember a time when you've had a feeling something more was going on in a situation than met the eye, or you felt something was about to happen before it did. That's called intuition – knowing what feels instinctively true. It's deep and complex. Many of us lose touch with this gift.

When tuned in, our sixth-sensory trait gives us a strong connection to the subtle changes in our environment. If we've been culturally discouraged from trusting our intuition as we grow up, we ultimately disregard it. This can result in a disconnection from our whole being and our feeling bodies, which makes it difficult to trust our instinctual needs for proper self-care. Food and drink choices may slip or our sleep quality diminishes.

Highly Sensitive People

There's a cluster of traits defined in scientific research that shows some people have a nervous system that is biologically different. For clarity, the nervous system is made of the brain, spinal cord, sensory organs, and all neurons that serve as communication channels between various organs of the body. Traits are characteristics often determined by more than one gene. A set of sensitivity traits was first identified in the early 1990s by psychologist Dr Elain Aron, who pioneered research on an evolved trait she described as a highly sensitive person (HSP). According to Dr Aron, roughly 20–30% of the population think and feel everything more deeply due to differences in their genetic makeup and this affects how responsive their nervous system is. As a fellow HSP, I know it is not imaginary. We're wired with a nervous system that can pick up on more sensory inputs or not filter out various forms of stimuli as easily.

In mainstream Western society, there's a lack of understanding about the scientific underpinnings of a highly sensitive nervous system, as it's not considered a desirable trait. However, in other places such as Japan and Sweden, the sensitivity trait is more highly valued than in most Western cultures. For example, in 2022 an observational study by Japanese psychology researchers compared the resilience of their sensory-sensitive subjects to the control group and found they performed better in challenging times.

Having a sensitive brain doesn't imply having a defect. Quite the opposite, it can be a superpower when you know how to fuel and drive your sensitive brain well.

According to Aron and other researchers, sensory processing sensitivity is not a new trait. From the perspective of a primitive age, it's been a protective mechanism. It can be incredibly important to pick up on dangers around us, through emotional or environmental stimuli. Hearing, feeling or sensing social cues early on when something isn't right enhances our ability to alert or help others get away from danger. It is a gift many types of healers and nurturers have as they naturally care and can detect the emotions of others. So it was, and likely still is, extremely beneficial for human communities. Studies have also shown that around 100 different animal species have this trait.

Being a HSP, also referred to as an empath, comes with strengths and struggles experienced less often by people whose brains are genetically less sensitive. According to Dr. Judith Orloff in her book *The Empath's Survival Guide,* all humans have sensitivities, though some more than others. As one herself says, "empaths are emotional sponges who absorb both the stress and joy of the world. We feel everything, often to an extreme, and have a little guard up between others and ourselves. As a result, we are often overwhelmed by excessive stimulation and are prone to exhaustion and sensory overload."

Highly sensitive people who try to fit in with the status quo and ignore uncomfortable signals from their bodies can end up developing sensitivities to bright lights, noise, certain foods or chemicals. This can be exacerbated if they've experienced significant adversity throughout life, perhaps from physical abuse, serious health challenges or neglect.

Suppressing sensitivities or frequently denying you feel them can result in emotional overwhelm and overthinking, which in turn can lead to physical expressions in the body. Our digestive system is in direct connection with the brain through the enteric nervous system. It's the common link as to why many HSPs and empaths are more likely to have gastrointestinal distress if they don't eat foods that are right for them or if they ignore their gut signals. Irritable bowel syndrome, autoimmunity and hypoglycaemia are all very common stress-related conditions that are connected to mental or emotional causes. It's important to see the mind–body interconnections and refine this if we want to rebuild health. Chapter 5 will go into this in more depth, including information on how to support your nervous system.

If HSPs aren't managing their nervous system right, patterns of internalising their true feelings can happen. This results in behaviours such as people-pleasing, conflict avoidance, hiding and shrinking. An essential step in the path toward reaching your full potential is to become aware of these psychological blockages and to work through them. I've included a HSP quiz in the resources list if you want to check this trait for yourself.

Many of those I work with, don't realise how sensitive they really are, or that it's even a thing. They're conscientious people with a strong drive to do well, who thrive on the adrenaline rush they get from recognition of their achievements. When this is coupled with their daily rituals of socially acceptable stimulants (like coffee) that suppress their appetite, emotional highs and lows plus behaviours can be extreme. Trillions of cells inside our human brain and body are too often run out of the energy they need to function well. When our cells are starving on the inside, it manifests as uncomfortable moods, lack of focus or automatically reaching for something to "soothe" for the moment, such as salty comfort food, sugary processed carbs or that extra glass of wine.

Many of us operate on autopilot most of the time, repeating old patterns such as this "reach and soothe" behaviour when we're feeling low on energy or in a negative mood.

Let me ask, if something is not working for you, how would you feel if it was? Are you willing to unlearn? Unlearning is an invitation to question. Unlearning old patterns starts with questioning current patterns.

Kathy's Story of Unlearning

A few years ago I helped a 48-year-old woman named Kathy who had reached her limit of trying to keep up with years of stressful work and family issues as a single parent. She had been struggling internally with these issues though now it was affecting her external world, especially her confidence at work and socialising. I sensed from her gentle nature and the way she spoke about the types of places and things that overwhelmed her that she was a highly sensitive person but as she'd never heard of the trait we just focused on her main concern—weight.

No matter how "healthily" Kathy thought she ate, she gained weight and was exhausted even after sleeping. She had seen numerous doctors before me and knew something crucial wasn't working with the standard mantra she'd been previously told: "Eat less, move more".

Frustrated with herself she'd say, "I'm really trying. I can help others achieve their goals. But I feel like I can't do that for myself with my *own* health. What's wrong with me?"

I told her it was not her fault. For years we've been given the same message, reassuring Kathy that "It's the one-size-fits-all message that's wrong. It doesn't take our history, genetics, life-style or any hormone imbalances into account."

Current research tells us that achieving our weight is not as simple as the old view of calories in and out. Weight gain, especially in women of Kathy's age, is actually a common sign of hormonal imbalance if food choices or movement haven't changed. Kathy knew her high-stress levels were part of the problem with her weight gain but didn't know where to start. She was keen to look at her hormone levels and genes to see if there were answers there.

Among other markers, her blood work showed her fasting glucose levels were within range but fasting insulin was sky-high at 17. Continuously imbalanced blood glucose levels affect all our hormones, especially insulin. Insulin is a fat-storage hormone discussed at length in Chapter 5.

Let's then consider the protective function our fat tissue has. Fat adds a layer of protection for us as insulation from harsh cold temperatures, pain and periods of starvation. This is not the type of environment that most people face in our modern world.

Thankfully, the human body has access to an important protec-tive tissue – muscle. Kathy realised muscle loss she experienced in her last five years was another part of losing control of her health. Muscle is crucial for more than an attractive body composition. Skeletal muscle is our primary energy-burning tissue, providing protection and strength, both physically and emotionally. Physical strength gives you a sense of control and confidence. When you're strong, you feel like you can handle things better and make positive changes in life. Muscle growth taps into the expression of the energy potential within your body.

We all have a natural tendency to lose muscle as we age unless we regularly lift heavy things. Loss of muscle can make us feel all our sensitivities even more. Wonder how? Notice for a second – do you feel weaker if you slouch your shoulders and spine? Now if you stand up with your back straight or stand up tall do you feel stronger and positive? Adequate muscle holds the human frame in a naturally healthier state.

I've witnessed regular weight training to be powerful for adults of any age to build muscle, reduce bone loss and have so many other metabolic benefits. The boost in mental confidence through building muscle can be especially beneficial for highly sensitive people. If you're admiring someone's muscles or flexing your own, take a minute to consider the motivation could be just as much for mental or emotional health as physical. If lifting weights isn't appealing to you, other ways of practising progressive resistance using body weight can also help.

Indeed it did with Kathy, we identified some gene variants that set her up to be prone to shaking off those stress hormones slower, firmly holding onto negative memories and finding it harder to control herself around addictive foods. These are all of the genes you'll hear about in Part 2. Her gene test alongside the HSP quiz confirmed my initial view that Kathy was a highly sensitive person and until then she had no idea how this awareness could help her. For the first time in her life, she felt like it wasn't her fault. Her genetically sensitive nature in an overstimulated environment was a huge part of why she responded to stress and food the way she had in the past.

This process helped Kathy gain trust in building a lifestyle that was unique to her. She quickly experienced positive effects from targeted supplementation, strictly staying away from specific triggers and was more motivated to consistently practice several calming lifestyle activities discussed in Part 3. With better sleep and a clearer mind, Kathy's work leadership skills improved, which opened up more business opportunities. She began lifting weights twice a week, losing unwanted body fat and regained her confidence to socialise again through her overall transformation.

Finding a New Way

Many HSPs, even if they're unaware there's such a trait, eventually with age, come to know they need different ways to feel centred, confident and safe with others around – no matter what else is happening in life.

While I've discussed many challenges in having a highly sensitive nervous system, there are also many strengths and gifts when nurtured well. Among numerous other studies is one where researchers used functional magnetic resonance imaging (fMRI) brain scans to measure the brain activity of HSPs, specifically neurochemicals in areas related to strong internal experiences. The 2014 study found increased brain activation in regions associated with awareness, empathy, attention and action planning. Research is validating that some of these traits are powerful leadership strengths to have. Having someone who can bring rich insights, thoughtful choices and detailed focus for deep work in today's world of short attention spans can bring a wonderful balance to a group.

Understanding how unique our nervous system response is can liberate us in all sorts of ways: Health, self-expression and relationships. Being uniquely accepting of all parts of ourselves can ease our minds and bodies.

Identifying traits of an HSP or an empath gives your body a compass to help regain trust in the wisdom that lies within your body, which can then send a signal that there is safety again. Once one of the roadblocks to well-being is removed other steps can be added in.

Sometimes when you're going through a really hard time, you might feel like you are drowning and can't see a possible way out. I've seen in my clinical work that when there's significant trauma in a person's past, they commonly lack joy and happiness in their present life. Quiet time spent in nature can bring small moments of joy and peace to HSPs. The right places outside may bring opportunities for these positive emotions to come back into your life.

PART TWO — INTERPRET

This section will piece together your mind-body signals and interpret the underlying root causes by looking into specific body systems.

The foundation of recovery from adversity and a life with energy and ease rests in three core areas:

1. Digestion – restore cellular energy
2. Brain – fuel and rewire the brain
3. Addictive behaviours – notice triggers and reduce risk

Think of these three forming the legs of a stool. They should carry equal weight to be a stable and firm foundation. This stability will support your mind-body balance.

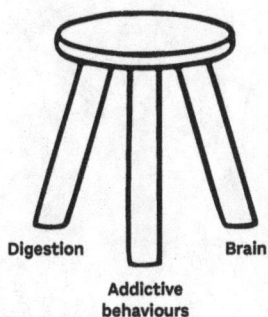

Digestion   **Brain**

Addictive behaviours

A field of study called lifestyle genomics researches the relationships between genes and lifestyle and how they affect our health and well-being. Lifestyle genomics can help us understand ourselves more accurately and guide us to make healthier and more beneficial decisions right up front. This awareness allows for better choices to reduce overwhelm or other factors that disrupt our body balance.

Researchers have identified the specific gene pathways that most impact our hormones, neurotransmitters, detoxification, metabolism, inflammation, cellular energy and mental health that overlap with areas in the overwhelm map. See Chapter 1 for a reminder of these areas.

This book focuses on nine priority genes that support behaviour change by optimising your brain and body function. However, other genes also highly influence your body's health defence, including MnSOD and VDR. If you implement the lifestyle, targeted supplements and food strategies found in Part 3, you will naturally support other highly influential genes not discussed in this book.

— 4 —

PRIORITY GENES AND SIGNALS OF DIGESTION

*"Everyone has a doctor within; we just
have to help that doctor do their work"*
— Hippocrates

Nutrient Starved Cells

The human body is complex but health solutions do not need to be. The foundations we are made of must not be overlooked. Addressing proper nutrition has played a vital role in improving human health since ancient times. In addition to what we eat, everything we think and do has an effect on our mind and body at a cellular level. It is all being recorded in our cellular memory. What we put in creates the quality of our cells that build the body and carry the mind. This accumulates into how we feel, look and act. When we interpret things from a big picture lens we can more easily see these connections.

Imagine for a moment that your body has similar needs to a beautifully designed, thriving garden. With sunlight, water and fertiliser, the plants grow enough to crowd out the weeds. The beauty and strength of living organisms increase all around the area you nurture, including deep into the soil.

When we mostly eat real foods, natural and unprocessed products we give our cells the ability to form the building blocks for strength, immunity and hormonal balance. If we get sick, a bit like when a storm hits our garden, we can bounce back faster or avoid developing new or rapidly declining health.

Eating highly processed foods is like starving good plants in our garden and feeding weeds. Without water, fertiliser or sunlight for plants, the weeds will take over.

At some point in time, without consistently getting the right fuel, the human brain and body have less cellular resilience and reduced ability to repair. In this situation, a diagnosis of a more serious condition than just weight gain or fatigue may appear to come out of nowhere, but it has built up over months, years or decades.

Prioritising our health can be a challenge when there is so much to juggle around us. All experiences in life can only happen through our bodies though. However, all we have is our body to experience life.

The human body is like a high-performance vehicle. Actually, it is the highest-performing asset we will ever have the privilege of having. Yet, through our food choices, many of us often put cheap fuel and nourishment into this high-performance vehicle. That might not be the case if we owned a luxury car or a private jet airplane. We would be required to only use the correct fuel so that it can function well.

When our body is resilient and feeling good we can take it for granted and start making poor nutrition choices because it can seem like we get away with poor fuel or nourishment. We continue to function, even if we are not functioning at our best. Ultimately, for our mind, body and brain to function the way we want to we have to prioritise the quality of food, not just the amount we put into our bodies. The higher the quality of food, the less toxin build-up there is and the better it makes us feel. In the long term, it means we're more likely to get the energy we want from that food and be able to sustain our functioning without having huge highs and lows in health.

Modern trends in eating low-nutrient processed foods, denying yourself food all day long or trying new habits like fasting, and then bingeing in the evenings, are unwise strategies. They will leave you frustrated by not being able to live with the vitality needed to function well in daily activities.

By understanding how your current state came to be you will see how a gradual build-up of foods and lifestyle actions have impacted how you feel. This will provide you with an opportunity to make different choices that powerfully change your body and mind.

Food For Your Microbiome

To illustrate how much our digestive ability can impact on daily lives, here is an example of someone I worked with.

Yvonne, 38, confidently walked into my office one summer. She appeared to be someone who took good care of herself. Within a few minutes of me asking what was going on and reading over her intake form, tears began flowing down her face. She apologised saying she used to be upbeat and fun to be around but was frustrated about feeling tired all of the time. The more helpless she felt, the more frustrated she would get, spiralling into what she described as a kind of "exhausted emotional stress." Her doc-tor suggested she try an anti-depressant to help her sleep more. Intuitively this did not sit well with Yvonne, so she was looking for other options.

She had been a sales consultant for over a decade, often trav-elling interstate on long road trips. Her hours had not changed. Her typical habits to recover were the same. Yet she was not bouncing back, no matter how many days off she had in a row. The more tired she felt, the harder it was to cook healthy meals or make good food choices while away from home. She did not have any obvious clues.

Alongside looking at typical foods she was eating, I suggested we start with a blood test to look for specific nutrient markers related to energy. I stressed to Yvonne, "The solution isn't just about which supplements could help you feel better, but asking *why* this is happening. Find and address the causes."

At a follow-up session, her results revealed a common pattern in women her age of very low iron markers, folate and B12 levels. She was eating red meat four times a week and was not bleeding heavily during her periods. This picture told me the missing puzzle pieces must be related to her digestive absorption.

When people like Yvonne eat plenty of vital nutrients but cells are not getting what they need, the cause of the gap needs some detective work. Were harmful bacteria "stealing" nutrients or blocking them from being taken into the cells? Did she genet-ically need a higher quantity of specific nutrients? Possibilities I considered were inflamed, damaged cells along the lining of her digestive tract, poor protein breakdown, gene variants or an infection. Once infection or parasites were ruled out, she invested in a gene test. While she was waiting for the results she started tracking the foods she ate with several symptoms. She quickly discovered some early clues by looking at patterns from a food and symptom diary. You will find a similar tracking diary in the resources list.

When her gene results came in, we discovered she had several genes that required support. Some gene markers are covered in this chapter. We could target ingredients in her supplementation and know why she might benefit from avoiding particular foods and strains of probiotics. Yes, that might sound surprising but not all probiotics are the same. In the wrong digestive environment, certain strains can make things worse.

I explained the overall cause of her food and energy level mismatch was due to her overall gut health, particularly cellular absorption and detoxification. With a better personalised understanding, she strictly took onboard the food timing and choices. I also suggested using the C.A.R.E. framework outlined in Part 3 along with two supplements and some lifestyle changes. Within two weeks her energy levels dramatically increased and within three months her sleep and mood patterns shifted into balance.

You have likely heard the old saying: "The way to a man's heart is through his stomach." For thousands of years, since Hippocrates' time in 440 BC, it has been understood that all disease begins in the gut. Being validated by modern science, mostly in the last 10 years, a major cause for that connection comes from tiny organisms living inside our digestive tract called the microbiome. Our microbiome is estimated to contain around 100 trillion living organisms (yeast, bacteria and fungi). In numbers like these, it is possible to see why we have as many of these organisms as we do human cells.

The microbiome influences not only our heart and digestion

but all organs of our body, especially the brain. The link with our mental health is through bidirectional communication between intestinal microbiota and the brain, known as the microbiota-gut-brain (MGB) axis.

You Are Made of What You Digest

Every single cell in your body depends on what you put into your mouth. Eating the right foods, at the right time and absorbing them well, can help you be physically and emotionally stronger.

All cellular energy and gene expression starts in your digestive system. All organs function based on the quality of raw materials in the form of macronutrients like protein, fats and carbs, plus vitamins and minerals you take in daily.

In a broader sense, what you take in through sight and sound in your environment also matters. It impacts your growth – either in a harmful or helpful way. It all accumulates and influences how you feel later. Sensitive people usually feel the feedback quickly, which means you are forced to pay attention. It is uncomfortable to ignore messages of discomfort for too long. Whatever you take in through mind and body impacts your whole being.

Try this mindful eating experiment if you want to see the effect.

- Observe or ask someone with you to notice what foods and how much you eat when you watch TV versus when sitting in good company and not watching a device.
- Do you eat a larger quantity of food or faster if you're watching TV?

Research in 2019 on grocery purchasing data assessed over four years revealed that over half (56%) of what Australians buy is ultra-processed foods. Many of us might be unaware of what defines food as ultra-processed.

One approach to identifying different foods is the Nova system, which groups foods according to their nature and extent of processing. The four groups of Nova classification are: (1) unprocessed and minimally processed foods (2) processed culinary ingredients (3) processed foods (4) ultra-processed foods. Ultra-processed foods contain numerous ingredients intended to improve palatability, such as food additives, modified starches and hydrogenated fats. Other additions rarely used in home cooking can include colours, non-sugar sweeteners, processing aids, emulsifiers, thickeners or gelling agents.

Examples of the most commonly eaten ultra-processed grocery foods include packaged bread, chocolate, confectionery, savoury packaged snacks, ice cream, carbonated drinks, cereals, ready-made meal sauces, margarine, dips or spreads, sausages, and burgers. All are harmful to long-term health and frequent consumption is best to avoid.

These processed foods and packaged takeaway meals are especially high in hydrogenated vegetable oils and starchy forms of sugar. They will build up within the body and lead to excessive inflammation. This accumulation affects the activity of our cells, which impacts our ability to have good physical function at every stage of life. The popular textbook *Wardlaw Perspectives in Nutrition* adds that adequate nutrient intake from food drives all cellular activity, either slowing down or stopping metabolic processes.

Filtering out Food Fads

The digital age makes it easier than ever to access food facts and opinions. But how useful or accurate is that information for us?

Consumer confusion is naturally high.

You have likely experimented with some food fads yourself – maybe some things worked for a while and others not at all?

Some governments create Food Guide Pyramids and distribute them through the medical system, attempting to cut through the confusion but their recommendations are often misleading and outdated. If you check the source of information there is often a financial link from agricultural, dairy or other food industries. Also, the types of foods and the way they are grown or processed have drastically changed, particularly since the 1850s. This was when the post-modern industrial food revolution began then further developed after World War II and even more since the 1970s. If you have not already, reflect on how your food is grown and produced. How much better and faster could you see positive personal health results if you were like a "food detective" with ingredients and food sources?

The food industry influences our choices by spending billions of dollars a year on social media marketing, promotions via diet "influencers", media, blogs and podcasts. Health advice today comes easily online, sometimes from unqualified attractive public figures who share their outcomes as, "It worked for me so it will work for you". Many claims are not based on large-scale studies, clinical experience or supported historically in the way ancient Eastern approaches are. It is remarkable how traditional Eastern medicine knew of nature-based principles about food and human health thousands of years ago. Many are still relevant to us today. Take an example of the current revival of using traditionally known ingredients such as bone broth and turmeric now used daily in many modern kitchens. Yet our ancestors knew of their benefits without testing them in a laboratory.

It's Not Just What You Eat But How You Eat It

I first met Marie when she was a single 32-year-old nurse. She had recently broken up with her boyfriend of two years. Desperately trying to get back in control of her life and health was at the top of her list. Recent emotional stress had made her menstrual pain and tummy problems unbearable. Confused with searching online for something to fix it all, she reached out to me for private support.

On her first appointment with me, I asked, "What did you have for breakfast?"

She replied, "I usually eat a pretty healthy diet. Today was my usual smoothie. Quick and easy to make then drink in the car on my way to work."

My eyes widened at the image of her "drinking and driving" in her car while heading to work. My surprised look was out of concern.

It is all too common. We live in a highly distracting modern world and many of us are not conscious of how we eat. I have been there too.

How often have you eaten a meal so quickly that you did not notice if you chewed each bite? Common habits like eating while looking at our phone or watching TV can creep in. Many of us are unknowingly getting far less out of our food than we should.

It is common to think that our digestion works so automatically that it will not matter. That is, unless we are in obvious pain, it all works normally. Though, as discussed in Chapter 3, what is commonly thought of as normal is not necessarily natural.

Irritable bowel syndrome (IBS) is the most common gastroin-testinal disorder in the world, currently estimated to affect around 15 per cent of the global population. It is a complex disorder of gut-brain interaction and not a diagnostic disease.

For many like Marie, it affects the quality of life, especially in stressful times. The most common symptoms are abdominal pain, changes in bowel movements and bloating. Stress causes abnormal functioning of the nerves and muscles of the bowel, producing IBS symptoms. A "dysregulation" between the brain, gut, and signal from the central nervous system causes bowel "irritation" or over-sensitivity to stimuli.

When noticing the gut-brain connection here you might see some parts related to how well one digests are within one's con-trol. This is not through willpower but starting with conscious awareness of your mind and body when eating.

Few of us think of our brains during digestion. This process actually starts in your head. The first stage is technically called the cephalic phase. Cephalic, means "relating to the head." It is for a good breakdown of protein and carbohydrates in food that is mostly forgotten unless you notice the subtleties.

As an example think of when you are hungry and watching others around you eat while waiting for your meal in a café. Your mouth might almost start "watering"? That is the natural production of saliva in your mouth, which releases enzymes to break down incoming carbohydrates. Experiencing gurgling in your stomach and properly chewing food stimulates the release of around a third of your stomach acid, or hydrochloric acid (HCL) that is essential for good digestion of that meal.

We are all born with this powerful natural substance which

should be as strong as battery acid in your car. Without strong pH (acidity) in the stomach, you will not properly break down protein-rich foods into amino acids. Which causes the food to putrefy. Yes, food can 'go bad' if it sits undigested too long in your intestines.

Good HCL also protects us from parasites and other harmful microbes. When HCL is weak or too alkaline the body is more susceptible to poor digestion, which can lead to reflux or an overgrowth of bacteria or yeast like candida that makes you crave sweet, starchy foods. These microbes signal to your brain what they need to survive resulting in cravings for sugars in any form. Contrary to popular belief heartburn is often a cause of too little stomach acid – not too much. Bacterial overgrowth in the small intestine interferes with your ability to break down and absorb nutrients from your food or supplements.

So if you want maximum benefits from what you put into your mouth think of where your mind is at that time. Eating in a hurry while distracted, walking or even driving will block a good amount of those digestive processes. It is best to slow down and take a short pause. Sit down, breathe, look at the food, chew it and give some attention to these micro-moments.

Strategies to Support Digestion

The following table talks through the stages of upper digestion, including what goes wrong and suggestions to support it.

Stage 1

When you see, smell or imagine food as well as when you chew, the brain sends messages along the vagus nerve (a cranial nerve that connects to your jaw and numerous organs), to tell special cells in your stomach to release acid (HCL). About 20 to 30 per cent of your stomach acid should be released.

What goes wrong?

Eating in a rush or feeling upset or stressed out, before or while eating, can block the signal from your brain to release enough HCL.

What can you do?

Turn down stress hormones or, if it is not the right time, wait a bit. It is best not to eat if you cannot focus on your food. Drink some water instead. When you can slow down to eat, take in a few deep breaths first and clear your mind before your first bite. Sit down, notice the sight and smell of the food then eat at a relaxed pace.

Stage 2

This stage is triggered as the stomach becomes increasingly full and amino acids are detected – about 50 to 60 per cent of stomach acid is released at this point.

What goes wrong?

Protein foods may feel heavier in your stomach if digestion is weak. Before working with me, many female patients were less inclined to eat much protein as they would interpret feeling heavy from protein, especially animal proteins, as a sign to avoid it. This is not the solution though – it is a clue that stomach acid (HCL) is low and cannot break down protein. A lack of bile from the liver may also cause inflammation along the stomach lining, this may then be interpreted as heartburn.

This often leads to antacid or other medication use, usually proton pump inhibitors which will further lower the body's ability to produce enough stomach acid. This sets up a breeding ground for an alkalising bacteria like H.pylori, causing further discomfort.

What can you do?
Take one tablespoon of apple cider vinegar about 10 minutes before meals (or with a meal, such as in salad dressing), and use herbal digestive bitters or a supplement like betaine hydrochloride. There are many foods to add and avoid, suggested in Chapter 8, which will naturally nourish the liver to regenerate and produce more bile flow. This will help protect the stomach lining and is essential for the lower part of the gastrointestinal tract.

Stage 3
When food starts to enter the small intestine, the remaining 10 to 20 per cent of HCL is released along with enzymes from the pancreas.

What goes wrong?
Insufficient enzymes will limit food breakdown which can lead to malabsorption and nutritional deficiencies. Fermentation and putrefaction of undigested food in the small intestine allow for an overgrowth of bacteria, especially when there are other motility problems.

What can you do?
Help the pancreas by taking a high-quality practitioner-brand digestive enzymes supplement to assist food breakdown and absorption. This is especially useful when eating out or having foods you are not used to. Brand quality varies so much that I recommend you seek professional advice.

Interpreting Gut Wisdom

Good nourishment comes not only from *what* you eat, as was mentioned earlier but *how* you feel – your emotions and thoughts – when eating. Your neurotransmitters, hormones and even blood flow all respond according to your state of being based on the surrounding environment. Gut awareness goes much deeper than the physical body.

Do you remember the first time you fell in love?

Or the last time you had "butterflies" in your stomach before a big presentation or performance?

The old saying "trust your gut" is more profound than just a sense you have without a concrete understanding of why.

Gut feelings are one physical manifestation of our intuition. So sensitive to our thoughts that scientists now call those "gut feelings" our "second brain."

Emerging research has validated that the connection between those physical signals and our intuitive sense is from a direct link between the microbes in our gut with our brain, termed the gut–brain axis. This is a bidirectional highway of information from the body to the brain and vice versa through what is named, the enteric nervous system (ENS). The multitude of nerve cells in our ENS allows us to "feel" the inner sensations of our gut (digestive tract).

The latest research shows we have more nerve signals coming up from our gut to the brain, about 90 per cent, and only about 10 per cent descending from the brain to the gut. Both positive and negative stimuli affect how our mind or body responds. This is core to the understanding of our mind-body connection.

The vagus nerve is central to the gut-brain axis, as it is the longest cranial nerve in the autonomic nervous system. Vagus in

Latin means "wandering" and this does that, connecting many vital organs with our brain. The vagus nerve carries about 90 per cent of our parasympathetic nervous system, commonly called "rest and digest" mode.

Our nervous systems do not distinguish between a real threat in front of us or something imaginary. For this reason, even watching something violent or stressful on TV while eating is going to have some effect. Avoid watching the evening news if you want maximum nourishment from your meals. Our emotional state, digestion, hormonal pathways and direction of blood flow are all closely connected through our nervous system.

Likewise, if you are in good company and feeling relaxed, your energy becomes more open and expansive. This allows your body to receive nourishment from the foods you eat and benefit far more from that experience. In the next chapter, we will more deeply explore the nuances of shifts in the state of the nervous system.

Epigenetics and Digestion

Epigenetics is the study of how cells control gene activity without changing the DNA code itself. This ever-changing influence comes from all our daily inputs. That is, all we can do to minimise risks and create a favourable outcome in health quality – mostly through frequent choices we make with our foods and lifestyle factors. We can have a significant influence over these. These factors influence our genes, which then give specific instructions to cells to function differently. Through this process our food eventually becomes the cells we are going to make and how we will feel. All physical health and mental states start with how our cells work. If we want to have a higher-quality mind and body we need high-quality nourishment.

Improving digestion is a good place to start when upgrading the quality of our inputs. Sometimes it is a simple upgrade like changing the way food is prepared. Do not dismiss the food itself. Such is the case for those who react poorly when eating excessive amounts of usually healthy foods like raw leafy greens in smoothies or salads. These are clues for a functional medicine clinician that there is a lot of damage along the digestive tract. To help make these foods less irritating to an inflamed digestive system, I will offer you some simple cooking suggestions in Part 3.

Think of food quality and lifestyle upgrades similar to software updates you can install on your computer. The upgrades of foods you eat and lifestyle habits will better align with the needs of your genes and lift your potential for things to work well. This will allow you to bounce back sooner from inevitable life challenges, however, when we do the opposite our risk for poorer outcomes goes up.

Drs. David and Austin Perlmutter, authors of *Brain Wash*, have coined the term "disconnection syndrome" which refers to the "modern disconnection with our DNA", meaning that we are eating foods that the human genome does not recognise.

For those who have inherited poorer detoxification ability or cellular energy, there are specific genes in priority pathways that can function better when they know how.

Three Priority Genes of Digestion and Energy

1. MTHFR – Your Cellular Energy and Detox Gene

Methylation is the critical biochemical process for every cell to function well by releasing toxins alongside repairing and making new DNA. How we make energy, respond to stress and how well our cells function or handle inflammation involves methylation.

Methylation is the process of transferring methyl groups to your DNA, which happens billions of times a second. A methyl group is made of one carbon and three hydrogen atoms. Methylation is vital to regulate our gene expression which, in turn, regulates increasing or decreasing cell function.

Methylation can help:
- DNA replication - vital for fertility and renewal of every cell in our body. The cells lining our digestive system are one of those, normally replaced every 4-5 days
- heal damage to cell membranes to get the energy to our cells
- regulate and clearance of hormones

To add methyl groups to our DNA (or take them off) our body needs adequate micronutrients. Micronutrients are the vitamins and minerals that help repair the usual wear and tear our DNA structures incur from daily living.

One primary pathway for the methylation process is activating the folate cycle. This pathway involves converting several essential B vitamins, which cannot be stored in our bodies, so regularly obtaining them from our diet in the right quantity is important. Rich sources of natural dietary folates are found in dark leafy greens, liver and some legumes.

Many grains are fortified with vitamins such as folic acid, the synthetic form of folate. There is evidence to show, however, that folic acid can inhibit MTHFR activity and be problematic for methylation. I recommend avoiding all folic-acid fortified foods, including bread, cereals and "health bars" or supplements with this synthetic folic acid added.

As mentioned earlier we are all born with a specific set of genes in our DNA and these genes cannot be changed. However, we can alter the expression of our genes by changing the inputs from food, lifestyle and our environment.

2. FTO - Your Satiety Regulator Gene

FTO was the first gene associated with obesity and remains the most significant. FTO is a nutrient sensory gene with the highest expression in the hypothalamus. FTO is also expressed in our fat tissues (adipose cells) and muscles. Recent studies have shown that FTO can control eating behaviours through satiety signals in the central nervous system, as the hypothalamus is the brain region important for appetite control and hormone regulation. FTO's influence on our fat mass and body weight is connected to not feeling satisfied after eating a meal.

There are several versions of this gene, AA, AT or TT – a gradient of variants, ranging from high obesity risk to lower obesity risk. The risk of obesity is thought to increase up to 70 per cent in those of us who inherit the AA and slightly less for the AT version.

According to some studies, people who carry the AA or AT variants tend to feel less full after meals, are more likely to eat when triggered by emotional cues, eat larger portions of food, and be more tempted by fried foods and sugary or fatty foods.

I have the AT version, so I am right there with you if you also have these temptations. You may be more likely to have habits such as frequently eating larger meals, seeking out seconds or wanting daily desserts or snacks which can make us easily prone to gaining weight.

Awareness of this gene and simple tips such as these may help:

- Limit portion sizes (use smaller plates and/or smaller forks) to trick your mind into feeling like you are eating more.
- Pace your eating. Eat mindfully and slowly by putting down the fork after each mouthful. Know that intuitive eating does not work so well for those with this variant.
- Frequently choose nutrient-dense meals as closely found in natural form.
- Weigh foods like protein if trying new recipes to adjust to the visual size of portions – types and quantities.
- To help feelings of satiety, eat adequate daily fibre from plenty of low-starch foods listed in Chapter 8.
- Avoid high GI, high-calorie foods – even if they are labelled as healthy foods like dried fruits, keto snacks and processed "health" bars.
- Limit takeaway or restaurant meals as a regular habit as you have less control over the cooking oils and added ingredients. Eating out as a treat or a special occasion is fine.
- Keep a food diary or track meals through a food app to help see how much and what types of food you consume in a typical day.
- Be consistent in making good choices that are visually tracked. Food education including reading and understanding food labels clearly can help.
- Create a new visual picture of the amount of food you need to eat at each sitting.

- Understand that higher levels of self-control will make this easier to manage. Enlist support from others to help watch meal sizes.
- Brush your teeth after meals to freshen your mouth and end eating time.
- Maintain regular exercise or movement.
- Check the ratio of waist to height (an indicator of metabolic health).
- Fast overnight for a minimum of 12 to 13 hours with only water. Eat only three main meals during daylight hours, with no snacking in between, to reduce overeating.

3. CLOCK - Your Sleep Timer Gene

This gene relates to our body's demands for sleep. Variations in this gene can harm our levels of ghrelin, the hormone that controls appetite, which is discussed in the next chapter. This gene variant can increase weight loss resistance by increasing hunger signals.

Many people with this variant feel the need to sleep for shorter lengths of time and prefer to be night owls rather than early morning risers. This is referred to in our modern times as a disruption in our circadian rhythm or sleep-wake cycles. This sleep routine does not align with the natural rhythms of daylight and darkness that humans were used to in ancient times. The consequences on hormone level concentrations such as plasma ghrelin can increase from lack of sufficient sleep, which often leads to weight gain. Around a third of overweight or obese people sleep less than six uninterrupted hours per night.

Awareness of this gene and these simple tips may help:

- Establish a regular sleep-wake cycle, particularly when going to bed late
- Minimise light and noise in the bedroom
- Ensure there are no artificial lights from radios, alarm clocks or any screens including phones
- Avoid exercise too close to bedtime (regular movement before 6 pm can be beneficial though).

Fundamentals

In my clinical practice, I have found most people are relieved to discover they had not previously been meeting the most basic needs of their cells, and thus, reflected in their results. Without the fundamentals in place, there is a limit on your full potential in body and mind. Remember, it is not about eating less food but getting enough of the right foods. In Chapter 8, you will have options to choose from in the foods to add lists and create meals based on your personal preferences.

— 5 —

PRIORITY GENES AND SIGNALS OF THE BRAIN

*Mental power cannot
be got from ill-fed brains*
—Herbert Spencer

Fuel for a Better Brain

When times are tough it is common to think that stress and poor mood are beyond our control and, therefore, solutions are too.

But the research begs to differ!

Given the right conditions, we can positively influence our quality of life to some degree.

Every single cell in our body depends on what we put in our mouth. At every meal or snack, we have a choice to start over and influence our physical needs. If we turn to our individual nutrition needs we need to appreciate that it is unique.

We are unique because of our biology, genes, lifestyle, and life stage. This is the complexity of individualised nutrition.

We have to appreciate that we may require more or less of certain nutrients than our best friend, partner or even ourselves at a different time in life.

Maybe if we had more sleep, worried less or had not discovered our favourite dark chocolate, things would be different.

Sometimes when I say this to people for the first time, it is met with disbelief. "Don't I just need to take something for my brain?" and "How could something as simple as what I eat every day be potent enough, powerful enough to change my mood? To have control of my thinking?"

The answer is this: Your brain is built off the back of the same nutritional building blocks that fuel the rest of your body. It is all connected, all made from the same stuff. It needs raw materials for it to function well. Those raw ingredients are the macro and micronutrients in the right quantities, in various forms of energy or vitamins and minerals from our foods. When our cells receive the nutrients they need, the brain also gets the signal that it has what it needs. Our psychology is thus supported by strengthening our body. Energy in our cells gives our biology strength. With better energy, we can improve the capacity of our brain cells to make new connections. We think more clearly.

Think of a time when this was not happening. Your daytime pressures were too much and you were undernourished or not eating well. It usually makes sleep more difficult. Poor sleep means less repair and toxins cleared from the brain. This cycle makes it even harder to make good healthy choices the next day or regulate emotions well.

You might even eat plenty of food and think, "Surely I am getting lots of nutrients from what I eat!?" But focusing on calories alone, rather than nutrients can lead to mixed messages for hunger in the brain. If you have a hard time feeling full, know there are two likely reasons at play – certain hormones and genes. The priority genes for digestion and cellular energy I will touch on shortly.

Firstly though we need to interpret messages driven by key hormones: Insulin, ghrelin and leptin.

Insulin

Insulin is the hormone that allows glucose into cells when all is working well. When cells signal they are full or not responding, excess sugar is stored as body fat. This is where long-term blood glucose problems can lead to conditions called insulin resistance or diabetes type 2.

To interpret insulin's connection with weight gain, let us consider a new way of thinking about it. In the earlier stages, insulin resistance or diabetes type 2 reflects an energy shortage – a deficit of energy production for the cells. Cells have trouble converting blood glucose into usable energy. High blood glucose does not equal cell energy. That is insulin's job – to allow entry for glucose into the cells. Energy-empty cells send other signals to help out the brain and body.

Ghrelin

Ghrelin is the main hunger hormone. When this hormone is out of balance, it can make you feel constantly hungry. I remember it as a "gremlin" when it is out of control.

When we regularly eat nourishing main meals with natural whole foods from plants, quality protein and good fats, our brain receives the signal that our energy needs are met and no more food is needed. If our meals frequently lack nutritional value or there are other inflammatory problems in the body, our brain will get this signal too. The response then is to secrete more ghrelin. The typical Western diet in our modern world creates a hunger cycle to keep us eating often yet hungry soon after. Ghrelin is one of the hormones signalling that message.

Leptin

Leptin is the third key player in this hormone symphony. It normally rises after eating a meal, telling your brain that you are full. It is nature's appetite suppressant. When cell receptors that should accept the signal become resistant (stop listening to the signal), leptin does not work as it should. Leptin resistance seems to have several causes and is an area of growing research related to obesity.

So often our inability to eat better or eat less unhealthy foods is not usually from poor willpower. Our hormones and genetics have an interconnected role. Different cells need specific nutrients, not just any old calories. Your brain is always sensing and interpreting your internal body signals to keep your balanced hormones and cells functioning. Certain genetic variations alongside hormone dysfunction really can compromise our ability to curb cravings – making us want to eat more food and not easily feel full. Our susceptibility to being tempted by ultra-processed foods goes right up unless we know why.

For the past few decades, the majority of the Western population deviated from our historical, ancestral diets. For example, many of us moved away from nutrient-dense high-quality fats (like butter, which is rich in vitamins A, D, E and K) and replaced them with harmful versions for our mind and body. These vegetable oils might be marketed as healthy but are actually very inflammatory, especially for our brain (which is made of more than 60 per cent fat) and lack those good soluble vitamins from natural fats like ghee and butter. When we miss those nutrients our cells respond by telling us to seek out more food and so we feel the need to eat more.

The same factors that can improve the health of your body, discussed in detail in Chapter 8, will likewise support your brain. Applying the right food and lifestyle interventions when early signs of disturbances appear in mood or behaviours can greatly reduce our risk of more serious degenerative brain conditions. Part 3 will detail how you can build a nutrient-dense diet, in a simple formula, that will naturally balance the hunger and craving hormone signals from leptin and ghrelin. I have seen successful results from using this numerous times.

Your Safe Vibes Detector

All humans have a biological need for social connection. It is how our ancestors learned to survive and build communities, helping each other and passing on stories to protect and warn others of danger.

I love the saying, "Connection is protection." That is, as long as it is a safe connection. Positive thoughts come much easier for all of us when our sense of physiological safety is met.

We are all designed to have the ability to pick up on the vibes or sense safety around us. Some vibes are easy to notice and cannot be ignored. Have you ever wondered why, without logical reasons, some people make you feel unsettled? Every moment we are alive, without conscious thought, we are born with the ability to assess for cues of safety.

We have a stone-age nervous system. No matter how advanced technology and modern medicine have become, humans are biologically wired to particular stress responses when confronted with volatile environments, unpredictable events and constant pressures.

Our ability to perceive subtle energy within us, emotional or physical danger from our environment is there to protect us. Our body takes it all in like a sponge and responds automatically, just like the functions that control heart rate, breathing and digestion. We would be unable to sleep at night if we had to think about our heartbeat or take each breath.

Professor of Psychiatry, Dr. Stephen Porges coined the term neuroception in his research to describe our brain's process of evaluating risk without conscious awareness. His research introduced the discovery of the *Polyvagal Theory* in 1994 as an updated explanation of how our nervous system works, related to how our body handles emotional stress and social connection. Polyvagal explains the essence of our social behaviours, how we can get stuck in maladaptive modes after trauma and what can be done to resolve long-term disruption of human connection.

Dr Porges focused his attention on the vagus nerve, which is the longest nerve in the autonomic nervous system (ANS). As mentioned in the previous chapter, the vagus nerve connects the mind and body as a two-way communication pathway between our digestive system and our brain.

Back when I was in college physiologists taught, and some are still (incorrectly) teaching that our ANS has only two states – sympathetic (fight or flight) and parasympathetic (rest and digest). The vagus nerve is the main component, transmitting about 90 per cent of the parasympathetic nervous system. Dr Porges' research discovered a contrary theory that we have three states, the third being freeze. These three states form a hierarchy (similar to climbing a ladder).

Our energy levels shift along with our ability to connect with those around us, depending on the internal signals perceived, like changing gears in a car – shifting from acceleration to brake or staying neutral.

Every day we move through different states in our nervous system, usually without awareness of this connection to the responses in stress hormones, energy levels and sociability.

This perception shift based on the polyvagal theory can help us to interpret situations based on what we *feel* first (i.e. a bottom-up view), as separate from our thoughts, rather than just analysing *what we think* (i.e. top-down view) to find a solution.

Colours of traffic lights can be a guide to the three states we can experience:

- Green = relaxed – calm energy
- Yellow = fight or flight – high energy
- Red = shutdown, freeze – low energy

The immediate needs to help us move through each state are quite different too.

In the yellow state – sympathetic stress response – you need to feel supported. If we have to act on our own, we use a lot of adrenaline in the short term to overcome a situation perceived as "fight or flight". With the right support around us, we should move through this state faster, back to the green – relaxed – state.

In the red state – the shutdown and overwhelm response – you need to feel safe. We freeze and shift into our primitive dorsal vagal, parasympathetic state in which we have no energy and motivation. In this state, it is also hard to ask for help or trust new people.

In the green state – relaxed, secure and confident response – you can handle it. You are in the ventral vagal, parasympathetic state and able to trust others, and more easily connect socially. Growth and restoration of energy happen in this phase.

Two main reasons we get stuck in a yellow or red state are:

- Too much too soon. The stress load is too big to handle.
- Too little for too long. A lack of support, care or even lack of physical nourishment to fuel the body has left you empty of any strength.

One of my favourite clinical tools is the *Polyvagal Flipchart*, created by Deborah Dana. I use this flipchart to give those I work with a visual of the three polyvagal states (also called the autonomic ladder). Simply put, Dana states, "Resilience is an outcome of being able to flexibly move up and down the three states in the automatic ladder many times a day." So it is normal to alternate between these states but we do not want to get stuck in "yellow" or "red" states.

If we are regulating well, this feedback will give us a sense of security by instantaneously and accurately reading signals in the environment. We detect and respond to a situation in front of us based on others' facial expressions, gestures and voices. We continuously send out subtle and obvious signals through our eyes, volume and tone of voice. It can give us the confidence to trust ourselves, take cues to relax or eat and filter the feedback from others who feel safe for us to engage with.

But if we are not regulating well, it is a different story. Think of it as being similar to having the latest high-quality home security alarm. If it has been tampered with or an intruder has tripped a wire and the system has not reset, it can stay stuck in that mode. Your alarm system might turn up the volume and intensity for numerous internal reactions, even when things are quite normal around you. This is why being stuck in dysregulation can get in the way of our quality of life and relationships if left unresolved for too long.

After extreme or chronic stress, the accuracy of this inner awareness system is faulty and often sends us the wrong message (telling an inaccurate story about someone around us, about our-selves or our environment). This is because we feel stress before we consciously think of it. A dysregulated system (from unhealed trauma) can misinterpret signals of danger when this may not actually be accurate. If you have inherited traits of sensitivity and have also experienced significant traumatic adversity this can create a more finely and tightly wound nervous system.

Traumatic life experiences shape our innate need for social connection, shifting us into unconscious modes of protection and constant self-regulation. While this might seem like a strong, reliable strategy, it is not. It affects how we feel, behave, trust and connect with others. While we do not always want to rely on others to help us, and to know this world can be a safe place, we need to know others are there if we need help.

Being in a mode of too much self-regulation a prolonged sur-vival response in sympathetic or the yellow state, there is limited safety for healing and human connection to occur. Healing means to "return to wholeness." Wholeness is not only within our minds and bodies, it also refers to feeling part of our collective society.

Unfortunately, feeling like we can do it ourselves in the wellness world is even easier in our modern internet age. The problem with self-diagnosis, using "Dr Google" for answers to symptoms, is that it often leads to confusion about treatments and an inability to admit we need help from other people. Yet all humans have a biological need for social connection. Remember, there is protection in connection with the right people. Being able to ask for help is a true sign of health, trusting that our world is safe.

To befriend our nervous system, we need to know how to interpret the state we are in so we can quickly intervene and regulate again. Simple resets on our nervous system are often the starting point, flicking the switch back to a signal of safety and calm to the body. Wheels are in motion for progress when our brain's primitive need for safety and survival has been met. The body can then relax and take care of the next steps.

Knowing where we are on the polyvagal map can help interpret your autonomic nervous system better. It can bring a sense of organisation to our states that can reduce that out-of-control feeling and reset to regulate again. It gives language to make it easier to explore new experiences, and to trust ourselves and others again.

Struggles Behind the Surface – Heidi's Story

I emphasised to Heidi: "Your reactions at the moment are not a reflection of who you truly are. You cannot use positive thinking alone. If your brain is starved of the right ingredients, your cells and genes are not getting what they need to work well. So your body is sending signals for help via those gut pains and stress hormones."

One of the easiest things Heidi took onboard to fix this was my suggestion to use her phone alarm as a reminder that she needed to eat at fixed times. She was not allowed to skip meals. Three evenly spaced meals every day between 9 am and 6 pm.

She followed the lifestyle and food guidelines of C.A.R.E. – that we will get to in Part 3 – and within a week she felt a lot less pain and anxiety. Within 12 weeks she felt more calm, balanced and happier than ever.

Sometimes we try to normalise our stress responses when we cannot manage or control how we feel. Recent research shows that those people with high sensory processing sensitivity (using the HSP scale) can experience a greater intensity of this perceived stress.

All our neurotransmitters are chemical messages in the brain, made from essential amino acids. When our diet lacks sufficient protein we cannot adequately rebuild crucial brain chemicals to think and feel good. When we tax our nervous system too often our brain detects this as a danger or triggers a trauma response, flooding your system with hormones like adrenaline and cortisol. This happens even though potential 'threats' do not only come from our external environment.

Every human brain needs a steady blood supply of oxygen and fuel for energy. Although the brain only accounts for only 2 per cent of your body weight, it consumes 20 per cent of your daily energy.

The brain's main energy source comes from glucose, though under specific conditions, it can use ketones from the breakdown of fatty acids. The brain does not store glucose like the rest of our body. When there is a lack of fuel supply available to the brain, our amygdala may perceive a survival threat. The amygdala is the brain region that senses danger, which then stimulates intense emotions, such as fear and aggression. This detection sends a signal for our hypothalamus to respond. The hypothalamus, also in the brain's limbic system, intersects our nervous system with the hormone (endocrine) system.

A cascade of hormone changes then sets off to impact and influence how we feel and behave. These signals from our hypothalamus increase our heart rate, blood sugar and blood pressure. They regulate our emotions, sleep, hunger and body temperature. If you are genetically wired to have a slower recovery (you clear hormones slower from your body) or you perceive stress at a higher intensity then excessive stress can be detrimental. Studies show that if you have prolonged levels of stress hormones in your system this can damage DNA and promote inflammation through releasing cytokines (chemical messengers). Without the right treatments, you can keep feeling stress even when there are no immediate threats.

Heightened stress reactivity often occurs in people with anxiety, depression or posttraumatic stress disorder (PTSD) and is strongly associated with certain variations in gene pathways for stress hormones (key genes discussed shortly). This all means that with prior genetic awareness, there is an opportunity to intervene before stress overload takes over.

I have observed for many people like Heidi, their symptoms are most often related to what is missing in the body and thus their brain. Our biology drives our behaviour and thinking. Biology comes from the Greek words bios, meaning life, and logos meaning to study. Together these words mean the study of life, which defines laws governing how living things interrelate, both physically and emotionally.

Here is an everyday example of how biology works to make it easier to understand what it takes to create better thinking and behaviours. Let us think of brain pathways as similar to hiking trails. A well-worn path becomes flattened and matted every time a hiker walks over it, just as when you fuel the brain differently, you can strengthen brain pathways. It takes time though. Changing what we eat or our habits for a few days is not going to make it solid and lasting. Over months and years of consistently travelling along the same hiking trail that is when it becomes a well-worn path. Efforts are worth it once new brain connections are made. You then have an easier ability to focus on better thoughts, feelings and behaviours with repetition and time.

Gifts and Challenges of Hypersensitive Brains

If you are a HSP, you are inherently different to about 70 per cent of the population, so trying to emulate the mainstream lifestyle may not align with your mind and body needs. If you follow *your* lifestyle design rather than trying to fit in with the norm, the beautiful gifts of being a HSP or empath can shine stronger without taxing your energy.

HSPs are naturally intuitive but after intense life challenges and when our gut and mind do not feel right, many of us feel blocked from using them. Maybe you do not trust intuition or feel unable to discern its accuracy.

Also, I often hear people say, "I do not know what are mine versus someone else's emotions." There are biological reasons why the emotions of others feel contagious to some of us. Whether positive or negative, emotions are all energy, moving something in us. The word "emotion" comes from the Latin word "emotere", which means "energy in motion". Specific brain regions and gene markers related to emotional perception have been identified as working differently in highly sensitive people and empaths.

Mirror neurons are a group of specialised brain cells that enable us to mirror the emotions we see in others. These brain cells are thought to be part of why HSPs and empaths often deeply resonate with the feelings of others. Judith Orloff, in her book *The Empaths Survival Guide*, says, "Our brains are wired for greater attunement with highly responsive mirror neurons".

Three Priority Genes
Affecting the Hypersensitive Brain

1. ADRA2B – Emotional Sensitivity Gene

A deletion of the gene ADBRA2B can account for differences in our emotional perception. The ADRA2B gene influences the hormone and neurotransmitter, norepinephrine, which influences our brain's ability to process emotional information.

If you have this gene variant in ADRA2B, the positive side is an increased predisposition towards making empathetic decisions. You are someone who can sense the emotional energy of others in a room. You intuitively pick up on body language and facial cues more than the average individual. Emotional intelligence may come intuitively to you, so you naturally build stronger emotional connections in relationships with friends and family.

This variant comes with a vulnerable side though. Decreased desensitisation of noradrenaline can result in a more vivid memory of negative emotional events such as arguments or fights. This can increase the risk of struggling with PTSD, especially if the trauma happened during childhood or includes significant physical or mental trauma. Having such a vivid perception of negative memories will make you more likely to avoid situations that could repeat or remind you of past negative experiences. If you often replay negative events in your mind, you might have a harder time letting go of things. You may need longer to calm down and return to a relaxed state.

A 2018 meta-analysis of 16 published studies, a total of 2752 participants, showed that those with the ADRA2B variant deletion had much higher perceptive ability and cognitive task performance when given emotional stimuli. Simply put, when these people were shown emotional images they had a more sensitive response than those with the intact gene variant.

The ADRA2B deletion variant was previously found to play a role in the formation of emotional memories, however, the new study shows that it also plays a role in real-time perception. In 2013 the University of British Columbia performed a study with 200 participants who were shown positive, negative and neutral words in rapid succession. Participants with the ADRA2B gene deletion variant were more likely to notice negative target words than others, while both groups were able to pick out positive words better than neutral words to an equal degree.

If it comes to light that you also have the ADRA2B deletion a stress-relieving lifestyle, foods and support offered in Part 3 are a must for supporting this gene and its pathways. Having a trusted reliable support circle can provide an outlet to share your feelings, rather than bottling things up and consuming you.

2. COMT –The Stress Clearance Gene

COMT (catecholamine methyltransferase) is a highly influential gene in pathways for our behavioural traits, gut-brain responses and hormone functioning. Its main role is to clear catecholamines (stress, reward and mood-regulation hormones), which are the neurotransmitters like dopamine, epinephrine and norepinephrine (adrenaline).

COMT is also a key enzyme affecting oestrogen clearance. It

is found in many organs of the body such as the brain (as neu-rotransmitters), liver, kidneys, gastrointestinal tract, skin, red blood cells and possibly in bone – so it is everywhere really.

Variants in this gene affect how fast or slow it works. These differences in speed influence our behaviours and how quickly we clear stress hormones from our bodies.

Slow COMT

Slow COMT can lead to a state of higher anxiety levels, low mood, increased adrenaline levels (under stressful situations), higher blood pressure, insomnia and more pain sensitivity or possibly migraines.

If you are a person who is highly driven and motivated, gets a lot of stuff done, but can become irritable quickly if out of bal-ance; and regularly struggles to stay or fall asleep, you probably have slow COMT.

Fast COMT

People with a faster COMT tend to be more relaxed, active, out-going and adept in stressful situations.

If you have a hard time focusing and others think you are laid back, or you are easily addicted, tend towards depression, and often overtrain when exercising you probably have a faster COMT gene.

3. BDNF - Brain Cells' Fuel Gene

BDNF is an important gene involved in the formation of new brain cells and the strengthening of existing ones. It acts like a "brain fertiliser", nourishing the cells and helping the synapses (connections between brain cells) grow.

BDNF is also a neurochemical found in the hippocampus, cortex and basal forebrain. All these brain regions are vital to mood balance, sleep and eating cycles, learning, memory and higher thinking.

Studies have shown that higher levels of BDNF make it easier for people to learn new things. Creativity and imagination are part of what helps humans adapt to change and these brain-stimulating activities help increase BDNF levels. Our brain cells can stay stronger, helping us become smarter and more neuroplastic (adaptable) even with age when we have higher levels of BDNF.

Lower enzyme function of BDNF is often associated with an increased predisposition towards repetitive thinking patterns and tendencies towards more feelings of irritation or frustration.

Adverse chemical toxin exposures and other stressful events in early life can negatively impact our DNA and change the expression of BDNF. This has the potential for a long-lasting impact on behaviour, memory and mood. Research studies in 2015 and 2016 on depressed adults found associations between reduced BDNF expression and serum BDNF levels.

Exercise and meditation are both activities shown to increase BDNF gene expression. A study in 2013 showed that just 20 to 30 minutes of exercise increased BDNF in the blood by 32 percent.

Knowledge Can Be a Motivator

Too often we are unable to see how our experiences and symptoms are related. When you make the connections, the healing momentum for recovery in both body and mind can transform into growth and strength. You will know how to better interpret the subtle signals of your body and see when you move between the different phases of the polyvagal ladder.

We have been focusing on interpreting clusters of interrelated genes and their metabolic pathways in Part 2, to help you understand how to best support them in a sequential order in Part 3. Think of this as a cumulative effect – it all adds up.

I have seen many patients benefit from insights gained in their genetic profile. Improved clarity and confidence came from knowing how to best look after their health: physically, mentally and emotionally. This health confidence has led to improved social connections, both personal and professional. Happy people regularly show up better around others.

Motivation comes naturally when you know the potential to make a difference in your genes lies within you. Waiting to be unlocked through focused efforts.

— 6 —

PRIORITY GENES AND SIGNALS OF ADDICTIVE BEHAVIOURS

"The dose makes the poison"
— Paracelsus

Freedom of thought is something many of us value. What we think and believe, affects how we feel and our outlook on life. These thoughts affect our everyday choices, from what we eat and drink, to our commitments with family, work or other opportunities. Things we enjoy, and people we find ourselves involved with at different times in life, can shape our habits.

It is natural to have a mix of both "good" and "bad" habits. What divides these habits and behaviours is seen in the results. Some impacts are minor while other behaviours can spiral out of control, with disastrous consequences.

Struggling to Unhook - Rose's Story

Too often I see capable, intelligent people who know their actions are harming their health, relationships or work, yet struggle to change them. There is much temptation in our modern world and without awareness, our genetic vulnerability can easily get us hooked when exposed to highly addictive substances.

Rose, 39, was someone I worked with who had struggled with yo-yo dieting for decades. She was a very driven woman, married with two kids and a successful media business. Her story to me revealed she was also a highly sensitive soul who had some unhealed childhood wounds. Despite Rose's stunning appearance, she lacked confidence in her looks and an excessive focus on 'fixing it' was exhausting her – easily triggered by others' negative emotions.

As a child, she binged daily on highly processed foods to comfort her sensitive soul. In her late teens, Rose began drinking alcohol every weekend, as she said, 'to relax her nerves'. Her vices further evolved as an adult into using cocaine with her friends at parties. She had tried to ignore the problems for years and avoided getting professional help until things reached a peak (or rock bottom?). Her marriage was an emotional roller coaster; she had regularly beat herself up for harmful, impulsive choices she would make and it was a spiral further affecting her body shape, moods and sleep. In an attempt to find a solution, her online search had led her to read about terms such as 'dopamine rush' and traits of an 'addictive personality' linked to genetics. Eventually, she made her way to my practice. She took her DNA test sample at her first appointment. By trying something personal and new to her Rose hoped the test insights could help her break free from the harmful cycle she was in.

In the weeks waiting for her test results I met regularly with Rose to help her understand the behaviour change that results from taking mind-altering substances are caused by massive shifts in dopamine levels in her brain. I wanted her to stop telling herself it was her "lack of willpower" problem. Excessively high dopamine surges change the stability of our brains and make us anxious, depressed, irritable and prone to making poor decisions when levels drop. With little or no impulse control there is less ability to care for ourselves or others.

The first defensive mechanism to keep addiction alive is denial of the problem. To avoid letting others know, hide the habit, behaviour or substance. For Rose to reach out for support and admit there was a problem was a turning point, a true act of courage. I wanted her to congratulate herself on taking this step towards positive change. She felt validated and relieved to hear this. You will hear more about Rose's recovery experience later in this chapter.

Addictions are a major obstacle for a freedom seeker. "Really?" you might say. "Don't we have so much freedom in today's world?" Yes, there is so much choice at our fingertips. The variety of foods and drinks we want are available almost anywhere, at any time. But ask yourself, are you choosing them of out of free will or being driven by a compulsion or urge that feels impossible to control?

Deeper meanings of a word can reveal its power. Addiction comes from the Latin word, *addictus*, meaning to be enslaved or bound to. There is an ancient Roman myth of a slave named Addictus, who was set free from his master's painful chains after many years of repaying debts. But he had become so used to chains that he wandered the land with his chains still attached, even though he could have removed them at any time. The relevance of this myth to modern addictions is a useful metaphor. For the addicted brain, it is about the shift in choices that can potentially kill them if left untreated.

Research has shown that addiction is a disease that chemically rewires your brain, making a person a "slave" to a substance or activity. In the addicted brain, the activity plus changes in biochemistry and several brain circuits affect pathways involving reward, stress response and self-control. Food addiction specialist and author, Dr Joan Ilfand, states, "Addiction pulls blood flow away from the neurons in the frontal lobe of the brain and that is where you make decisions and do problem-solving!"

It is not a lack of willpower at all. Every decision that person makes is hijacked. Rewiring the brain to its normal function often takes quite some time, patience and support – even after a person has stopped using the substance. Addiction separates a person from the true feelings in their body.

Addiction is both a physical problem and a cognitive dysfunction due to a person's psychological dependence. When a person becomes chronically and compulsively controlled by taking psychoactive substances (sugar, ultra-processed foods, alcohol or drugs), they cannot recognise their own freedom.

Types of Addiction

Every choice you make is shaped by how your brain regulates your body's basic functions. Every minute you are alive your brain is interpreting and responding to everything you experience in your environment. When there is a disruption of the normal, healthy functioning of organs in the body, such as the brain or heart, both will lead to seriously harmful effects.

Chronic brain disease is just as serious as heart disease. If left untreated both can last a lifetime and lead to death. Both are progressive, meaning they get worse over time but in many cases with the right awareness, actions and support both diseases can be preventable and treatable.

Addictions can take on different forms and a wide range of severity. The forms can be - substances we take into our body (intake addiction) that produce dependence, including processed foods, sugar/flour, alcohol or drugs – or excessive behaviours (process addiction) ranging from gaming, screens, gambling and sex addictions.

Addiction could develop from excessive gaming on your phone or from overusing socially acceptable substances like ultra-processed foods.

According to psychiatrist and author of *Dopamine Nation*, Dr Anna Lembke, four Cs alert us to behaviours that are potentially addictive:

- control (loss of)
- compulsion (automatic use)
- continued use despite adverse consequences
- craving (mental, physical or both).

Addictions are chronic, meaning that they will not go away on their own, and progressive – meaning the impact and use worsens over time and can be fatal if left untreated. Constant support protects someone from relapsing patterns, and the right environment is needed to restrict availability.

Differentiating between use that is normal, harmful or a full-blown addiction can be useful. Start by asking a few questions:

- Do you feel like you have control over this use?
- Can you consciously stop the substance or behaviour when you try?
- Is it harming other areas of life like finances, relationships or work?

When there has been repeated failure to resist a strong impulse, drive, or urge to repetitively perform an act or take something that overly rewarding effects bring about distress or interfere with your function or others around you, it is likely to be an addictive behaviour.

If you answered 'no' to questions 1 and 2 above, and 'yes' to question 3 I urge you to seek professional support. Global support groups can be found in the resources list.

What Predisposes Someone to Addiction?

In our society today, it is easy to normalise our vices. We all form habits to self-soothe or lift our mood and energy. Almost everyone drinks alcohol or caffeine in some form. We are all busy with the demands of modern life. When we are tired and want something easy to feed ourselves or our family it is normal for many of us to reach for easily accessible, ultra-processed packaged foods or takeaway. How much and how often we use them will influence the degree of harm they might bring us. When we can't live without them it is worth considering why.

Often overlooked is that some of us have very sensitive brains and risky genes that affect our neurochemicals when exposed to addictive substances. These substances can take control of our minds and bodies. The word *control* is the key.

Certainly, not all vices are addictions or even harmful. Healthy coping is great. It is controlled and empowering. Alarm bells should ring when addictive habits become disempowering and uncontrolled behaviours. Awareness is the first step to taking back control.

Addictions arise when there is a point that you want to stop the habit and you know it is not working well for you but you simply cannot. And when you do stop it, you feel negative consequences – physical or otherwise.

At least half of a person's susceptibility to addiction can be linked to genetic factors. Unless we are exposed as an unborn foetus to the substances, we do not usually inherit an actual drug addiction. We can however inherit genes that increase addiction risk sensitivity. Other influential factors are our environment and life circumstances, such as unresolved trauma, the culture we are brought up in, financial means, lifestyle habits, relationships and how we regularly handle stress.

The vast majority of genes are influenced by our environment, which then influences whether we express functions of these genetic risks or not.

Some people may have a high number (say 60 per cent) of risk genes but very little exposure to addictive stimuli, while others can have few genes (maybe 40 per cent) but much higher exposure. It is always a combination that decides whether something becomes an addiction or not.

Interpreting Connections Between Trauma and Addiction

Trauma and post-traumatic stress are much more common than people realise. It does not have to be from some extreme events. Any situation where you feel intensely overwhelmed and unsafe can trigger a trauma response where your system becomes flooded with adrenaline for too long.

In the short term common responses such as numbing out and dissociating can help us adapt to protect ourselves from feeling the full pain of the experience. Addictions are a common outlet for some of us to self-soothe the pain we have experienced from that trauma.

Other factors related to trauma and addiction include early childhood experiences of neglect or abuse or feeling constantly overwhelmed by being "too sensitive". A useful awareness tool – the Adverse Childhood Experiences test – can be found in the resources section and helps to get insight into your own risk of the effects of childhood trauma.

Risks in Running on Empty – Megan's Story

Megan reached out for my help when the loss of a loved relative triggered emotional stress. Unable to cope, she had become hyper-focused on her weight and appearance to regain some sense of control.

She was unaware that some things she was doing to lose weight were triggering addictive patterns. The constant yo-yo dieting, extreme exercise routines and long fasts were starving not just her body but her brain as well.

For most of us, our brains use glucose for fuel. Having prolonged weeks or months of very low blood glucose levels starves the brain cells of essential fuel, causing both physical and emotional symptoms. As discussed in Chapter 4, our brain does not store glucose like the rest of the body to quickly access it. Without regular, substantial, healthy meals our brain's critical blood supply can be interrupted several times every day. Once she understood why it mattered, Megan gave it a try. Within just a week she felt noticeably calmer, with naturally focused energy from eating this way.

Megan was also unaware that she was brewing the "perfect storm" by having a combination of many traits of a highly sensitive person and several high-risk genes predisposing her to addictions.

Now she knew *why* the food and lifestyle actions that I recommended mattered and were the vital pieces she had previously missed. She could now choose with ease to change unhealthy habits that would support her with living in the right-sized body for her by knowing how to work with her genetics. She liked my analogy that her brain was similar to a sensitive, sophisticated alarm system and by interpreting how to "drive" and "fuel" her brain well she had operated it better.

Addictions and Highly Sensitive People

Highly sensitive brains respond differently to dopamine, which is a neurotransmitter released by the brain when it anticipates a reward.

Researchers have found a connection between sensitivity (HSP traits) and 10 different gene variants that impact dopamine receptors. Other genes involved in high sensitivity such as COMT and ADRA2B, also affect how our body uses dopamine, discussed in Chapter 5.

Scientists have identified over 100 different neurotransmitters but monoamines are thought to be the most important brain chemicals. Dopamine is one of these monoamine structures along with serotonin, histamine, epinephrine and norepinephrine.

In a healthy brain, the right amount of dopamine keeps us motivated, focused and driven towards reaching our goals. It boosts our drive to pursue happiness, through actions promoting reproduction and survival (think sex and food).

In our modern world, this natural feedback system is often targeted by the processed food industry and large tech or advertising companies that keep us wanting more. Even coffee has anti-depressant effects by stimulating dopamine and serotonin, improving not only energy but mood as well – though it depends on how much of the substance we take. As the Swiss physician Paracelsus said 500 years ago, "The right dose differentiates a poison from a remedy."

Some Substances Are More Addictive

The harmful effects of substances on our brain's reward centre depend on how much dopamine floods in at a certain time. Excessive levels in a short time can lead to trouble with compulsive behaviours. Some substances and activities have a much greater mind-altering effect.

Dopamine increase of various substances, above baseline:
- Sugar–Chocolate   55-100%
- Video games   75-300%
- Nicotine   100%
- Sex   100%
- Alcohol   360%
- Cocaine   225%
- Amphetamine   1000%

For a brain that is genetically more sensitive to dopamine, due to gene variations, these amounts may be much higher. Our dopamine receptors are fragile to the damage from excessive production and can eventually lead to the death of dopamine-producing cells.

To prevent this damage from happening too soon, dopamine receptors will first down-regulate, making them less responsive. This is why an amount of a substance that once made us feel good can have less effect over time.

With repeated use, we end up in a dopamine-deficient state that does not feel good. That is an experience of pain and discomfort. Dr Anna Lembke, the author of *Dopamine Nation*, explains this is our brain's way of trying to bring everything back into balance and technically called homeostasis.

When we experience pleasure, dopamine is released in our reward pathway and the balance tips to the side of pleasure. The more our balance tips and the faster it tips, the more pleasure we feel. But here is the important thing about balance. It wants to remain level.

The extreme "highs" from certain substances and behaviours then tip the scales of balance by decreasing pleasure from other, more natural substances and activities.

Food Addiction

Just as not all drugs have the same effect on us, not all foods have an equal mind-altering effect on our brains. Some foods act like drugs in our brains. Most of us know our "trigger foods" – the bowl of steamed broccoli, usually is not on that list. Recent studies using brain imaging prove that sugar, flour and highly processed foods can act as psychoactive drugs on the human reward system, similar to the effects of alcohol and amphetamines.

Food addiction counsellor and author Kay Sheppard relates the intense brain effects to changes in our modern foods in her book, *Food Addiction: The Body Knows*, "All addictive substances start as natural substances, which are taken through a refinement process. These addictive substances are quickly absorbed, alter brain chemistry and change the mood."

Willpower is almost impossible when faced with an abundance of processed, refined foods and substances freely available. It is easy to see how so many of us can increasingly use food as a drug rather than a source of nutrition.

When struggling to break free from addictions to sugar or processed foods, imbalanced brain chemistry creates the uncomfortable withdrawal effects felt in mood and energy levels. The substance and addiction process triggers a dysfunction in our brain's reward circuit and affects our ability to regulate emotions and impulsive behaviours.

Diagnostic tools to assess food addiction such as The Yale Food Addiction Scale or S.U.G.A.R. (that stands for Sugar Use General Assessment Recording) can be useful to take out any guesswork for those in doubt. Links to these can be found in the resources list.

When we are ready to make changes it is never enough to just know that we need to avoid the trigger and then stop it. Creating balanced brain chemistry and recovery requires the right fuel to support our genetic predispositions.

Balanced Brain Chemistry is Crucial for Stability

We live in an overstimulated world where our brain has to filter all sorts of triggers vying for our attention or emotions. Unfortunately, this overload has worsened since the global pandemic of COVID-19 was declared in 2020 with lockdowns, health concerns and financial stress for almost everyone. This resulted in a massive rise in addictive substance use, especially alcohol, as was seen in surveys and studies about this topic.

To make rational decisions we all need a well-functioning prefrontal cortex. That is the area higher up in our brain that keeps our emotions in check and drives executive function for better long-term planning. This area only makes up one-third of our brain and has evolved over a very long but also quite recent time in human history. MRI scans have revealed the prefrontal cortex is most active when considering long-term consequences and planning for our well-being and that of others.

To create and maintain willpower and normalise brain chemistry, the prefrontal cortex needs an adequately stable supply of glucose. Unstable swings from high to low blood sugars cause drops in the glucose energy supply to the prefrontal cortex. This low energy supply also results in a surge of adrenaline and other stress hormones, which further impair effective signalling to the prefrontal cortex. It is part of the reason that research in the book, *Brain Reset* shows "the more continually stressed we are the more easily addicted the brain can become."

This stress response and lowered rational thinking reduce our ability to use our skills to protect our freedom, create recovery and say "no" when tempted by a trigger. It easily stimulates the habitual response towards using addictive substances and behaviours. On the flip side, a well-fed and balanced brain allows us to make good choices.

When the prefrontal cortex is off duty or "starved" of the required fuel, the main area that takes over is the amygdala. Our amygdala is the survival detector and is always ready to notice signals for fear and worry, which I discussed in Chapter 5. We cannot make rational decisions or better health choices from our amygdala, no matter how good our intentions are. It is a vicious cycle, where we keep making poor decisions because our brain's fear centre is dominating.

Hopefully, now you can see the reasoning behind why an undernourished brain is likely to make poor decisions – we lose impulse control and regulation of our emotions. So it is no wonder threats of fear and worry have our full attention and mental focus.

What Sets the Addiction Stage?

Remember Rose, whose story started this chapter. Her DNA testing results confirmed she had several gene variants that would greatly influence her addiction risk. This set her up to have a super-boosted response of dopamine when taking certain substances. The powerful psychoactive substances made her brain chemicals peak and then crash to the same proportion once they wore off. Her brain responded to sugary and ultra-processed foods in a similar way to hard drugs.

She had inherited a low baseline level of dopamine and thus her receptors were extremely sensitive to high-impact substances. This made her even more vulnerable during emotionally stressful times because her ability to handle chronic stress relied on the same neurotransmitter pathways. Her default habit to soothe stress pains had been to consume excessive amounts of fruit, fruit juices and even some processed foods labelled as "healthy" like gluten-free products. These were short-term emotional fixes that did not help her genes or cells function well. Her habit of skipping a meal every day and fasting for two days on weekends was especially harmful to her brain. Her brain was not metabolically able to use fat or ketones as its main fuel source, so glucose crashes made her moods bad. I suggested that fasting overnight for 12 or 13 hours was a natural rhythm but any longer was not right for her at that stage.

This interpretation connected the dots for Rose. Food addiction research solidly shows that skipping meals can be a primary trigger of the relapse of many addictions. When Rose ate high carbohydrate substances they brought on huge sugar surges, which subsequently resulted in low blood sugar crashes. The internal mental stress from hypoglycaemia (low blood sugar) affected her brain's ability to have rational thoughts to make good food choices.

Sugary drinks and refined grains have long chains of sugar molecules joined together, which can trigger addictive patterns in those who are genetically susceptible. In the addiction community, many forms of sugar are called the "gateway drugs for cravings". As the old saying goes, *"What goes up must come down"*. Our brain chemistry then changes to become wired to want that sugar fix again to feel normalised and reset.

Rose felt a huge relief knowing it was not lack of willpower that made her struggle for decades with rebound weight gain despite periods of intense exercise and food restriction. She longed to be free from her addiction and protect her mind from what she now understood was a brain illness. By healing her brain, her thoughts would become rational and she could regain control over her choices and life. With online support groups and my professional one-on-one support through sustainable food and eating style changes, supplements and routine activities she enjoyed, Rose escaped her addictive lifestyle.

Research shows that relapse is much more common in those who have fewer dopamine receptors in their brains. These people benefit from finding ways to feel pleasure from non-sugar foods or other non-drug-related rewards that still increase dopamine. Nothing extreme. Recovery requires adopting skills and new behaviours with the help of a supportive community.

Thankfully, several activities that support our nervous system, such as exercise and meditation, have been shown to increase the number of dopamine receptors we are born with. These details are discussed in Chapter 7.

Three Priority Genes Related to Addiction

Interpreting our priority genes that need attention alongside our body's current signals can become a powerful connection to lasting change.

Awareness of our gene markers will highlight potential tendencies if the right environment is not in place. They are a starting point, not the full picture. Full interpretation of other gene pathways (mentioned in previous chapters) that connect cellular energy, detox and stress response matched with your current condition and lifestyle will complete the insight.

Warning: Risk either in your favour or not, does not equate to a fixed reality. Even if you have none of these gene variations it does not mean you cannot become addicted to a substance. If anyone is continually exposed to something that produces epic levels of dopamine and has the means to keep using it there is still an addiction risk. This is what makes the availability of sugars and highly processed foods so problematic.

The following genes are closely linked to brain chemistry and risk for additive behaviours.

1. DRD2 – Addiction Seeker Gene

Pleasure-seeking behaviours, movement, desire, reward and motivation are feelings activated by the neurotransmitter dopamine.

A variation (SNP) in the DRD2 gene means there is a reduced number of dopamine receptors in the brain. With fewer places for this neurotransmitter to bind DRD2 affects the signalling of dopamine, thus a person needs higher dopamine levels to feel satisfied. Dopamine availability in our brain affects the drive or amount of effort we put into obtaining food and thus our behaviour patterns.

Have you ever wondered why sweet cravings are much more common than bitter-tasting leafy greens? The answer, you know now, is the sweet taste activates dopamine receptors in the brain which help us remember the experience and seek it out again. When you see your favourite ice cream or other sweet, and remember how good it was last time, dopamine levels rise and strengthen your desire for that sweet again. It does not matter if it is a lump of refined sugar or natural sugar, such as honey or dates – as far as the brain is concerned, it is all the same.

Having a variation in this DRD2 gene on its own does not mean the addictive trait is fixed, although when viewed in combination with other gene variants it does increase the risk of craving more desirable, highly palatable foods or other substances.

Ernest Noble, a biochemist at the University of California, in 1990 first connected a variant in a gene known as DRD2 with alcohol addictions. Variants in DRD2 affect how sensitive our dopamine receptors are and, thus how much dopamine can enter our brain cells. Dr Nora Volkow, director of the National Institute on Drug Abuse, explains in her popular 2014 TED talk based on decades of research that brain imaging studies suggest people with fewer DRD2 receptors are more likely to become addicted than those with many receptors.

DRD2 gene variants were first linked to alcoholism but since then it has been connected to other substances that flood the brain with extremely high levels of dopamine, including caffeine, sugar, recreational drugs, video games, cell phone use, online porn, gambling and high-risk competitive activities.

2. MC4R – Snack Attacker Gene
About 25 per cent of the population has this gene. This gene

produces the melanocortin receptor in the brain (our hunger centre) that signals the need to eat when energy levels are low. Once a person with this variant starts eating it can be difficult to stop. This person is more likely to have a disordered eating pattern and over-snack on products that increase appetite and decrease satiety. Research has shown a link to obesity among people with this gene.

3. MAO-A - Mood Swinger Gene
The MAO-A (monoamine oxidase gene) is responsible for processing the neurotransmitters serotonin, dopamine and noradrenaline. When functioning in balance these mood chemicals enable us to feel happy, calm and positive – or activate our survival responses to run from danger as well as our ability to learn. The gene MAO-A helps break down stress hormones and eliminate these compounds from our bodies.

Excessive stress triggers the production of higher amounts of noradrenaline and some dopamine too. This is why some people like persistent stress because it stops them from feeling depressed —they can be addicted to stress to lift their moods.

Extremes in lifestyle activity, from excessive exercise to being sedentary, negatively affect MAO-A. On the positive side research has shown that nature walks, regular sunlight exposure, qigong, meditation and yoga can benefit MAO-A regulation. Other supports for producing appropriate serotonin levels in the gut include omega 3s and the same dietary suggestions I will discuss in Part 3.

Gene variants can make this function either too fast or slow. Both gene types can exhibit addictive behaviours or overthinking patterns.

Slow MAO-A – the Irritable Insomniac

Slower enzyme function of this gene allows an excessive build-up of serotonin, dopamine and noradrenaline, as hormones are cleared more slowly than ideal after stressful events. Too much stress too quickly can cause behaviours like irritability, prolonged anxiety, aggression and mood swings as well as headaches, restlessness, trouble winding down and insomnia.

On the flip side, when people with this variant are not stressed out, they can be more productive, alert, focused, attentive, cheerful, self-confident and energetic.

When the activity of this gene (MAO-A) slows down many robust studies support a relationship between this variant and aggressive behaviours. Because this gene is found only on the X chromosome, men are more likely to manifest the effects of this variant if they have it.

Fast MAO-A – Hyperactivity and Anxiety States

A fast-functioning MAO-A gene will clear those hormones out quicker and deplete the brain of benefits. This can lead someone to often feel flat, bored, tired with depressive feelings and trouble staying asleep. To compensate for this they may seek out rewards and pleasure-based habits, from either carb or sugar cravings through to all sorts of other addictions – alcohol or gambling as well as other hyperactive behaviours.

Our genes influence behaviours and can guide us towards what occupations suit us most. People with fast MAO-A may gravitate towards things like higher intensity jobs such as hospital emergency care or risky occupations. These activities increase stress responses and make them feel more satisfied with the challenge. This type of person would be depressed doing an office job with low-pressure intensity.

Excessive long-term stress does, however, create more pressure on all our genes, uses up more essential nutrients and impacts on repair and numerous other bodily functions.

Behavioural Traits and Gene Variant Combinations

Researchers in the genetics field examine large population studies to explore connections between particular factors in gene variants and individual health outcomes or behaviours. Your behaviours are not just a random accident. Mood shifts are actually influenced by a combination of many genes interacting with your environment.

Gene Combinations Linked to Mood Swings

COMT and MAO-A: As the COMT genes share a metabolic pathway with MAO-A, having the slow enzyme variation in MAO-A can increase a tendency for mood swings, obsessive-compulsive disorders, aggression and other personality disorders.

MAO-A, COMT and MTHFR: When someone with this gene combination (MAO-A and COMT) also has a variant in MTHFR (your cellular energy and detoxification master from Chapter 4) it can give their brain lots of energy and focus as higher levels of neurotransmitters are available. At the same time, it can make it difficult for them to control their temper, rise above irritating situations or manage mood swings. These behaviour patterns can make it easier to reach for substances or behaviours to calm down, and make triggers for addictive patterns harder to tame.

Gene Combinations Linked to Metabolic Risks

DRD2 and FTO: When these gene variants are combined it puts someone at higher risk of overeating and addictive tendencies.

These together influence the risk for accumulation of body fat, insulin resistance, diabetes type 2 and dopamine-dependent learning traits. Namely not feeling easily satisfied from a good meal and learning to repeat the need for sweets afterwards, even when feeling full.

Gene Combinations Linked to Binge Eating

◆ *COMT (slow), DRD2 (high), FTO and MC4R:* The COMT gene controls how long you feel an emotion like pleasure and breaks down stress hormones. DRD2 controls how intense your pleasure response is. This combination of genes further increases someone's likelihood of using food as a coping mechanism for managing stress or negativity. There is a greater predisposition for either bingeing or 'risk-reward' behaviour patterns such as, "I have had an awful day at work. I need to reward myself with a tub of ice cream when I get home". Especially if one has not adopted other strategies to soothe emotional distress or is unaware of this tendency.

◆ *COMT, MAO-A and ADRA2B:* A combination of these variants is commonly associated with someone who may use food as a coping mechanism for emotional overwhelm or hypersensitivity. It can make someone more likely to identify with food or alcohol as a way to cope with, or escape from, stressful situations.

- *COMT, DRD2, and MAO-A*: These genes play a large role in our experience of pleasure in life. Excessive pleasure-seeking can influence inhibition, self-control and reward-seeking behaviours. This also may lead to an increased risk of chronic poor sleep, because addictive or bingeing habits related to food, technology or substances mean people are willing to forego proper sleep in favour of their pleasurable activity of choice.

- *FTO and MC4R:* The combination of variants in these two genes can lead someone to have more dysregulated hunger patterns. They may prefer to graze on snacks during the day, particularly at odd times. They may engage in "midnight snacking" or overeating, although they may not feel hungry if engaged in a consuming task that requires their brain to be engaged for hours with an achievable challenge and focused attention.

Heal The Brain to Protect Recovery

From Rose's story and insights into the priority genes discussed, you have likely seen connections between brain sensitivity, stress response and risk for addictive behaviours.

An addicted brain tries to stabilise itself and feel a new level of "normal" as the reward circuit pathways and neurochemicals tip to unnatural levels.

If a genetically addiction-sensitive person with variants in dopamine pathways frequently exposes their brain to substances that cause extreme dopamine levels, the seed of addiction is planted and can easily become uncontrollable.

It is very difficult to think, talk or read your way out of an addiction. So many people already know what to do but are unable to do it. This is because the brain chemistry needs to be reset for lasting behavioural change.

Sensitive brains need the right fuel just as much as avoiding triggering substances, along with psychological skills and support to rewire the brain to a stable natural state. Substance withdrawal without changing the fuel or brain nutrition rarely works long-term.

Food changes are hard though. If you address nutrient deficiencies by using a "food first" principle to meet this need then you have a lifelong approach to support your brain and make good behaviours stick. Taking on new eating habits can impact how we think, feel and act. When you gradually feel different, have better sleep, energy and more stable moods a "new normal" starts to take shape.

Unfortunately, many primary-care physicians and psychologists who work with patients suffering from various addictions lack an understanding of how to interpret genetic tests. The best approach is a combination. If you are interested in seeing your genetic profile, is worthwhile finding a qualified specialist who can interpret your test profile and also work alongside your addiction support team. See the resources list for further recommendations.

PART THREE — IMPLEMENT

Becoming aware of how we influence the environment of our genes we increase our chances of applying positive lifestyle changes. After all, awareness can be our greatest asset for change and is a fundamental tool for self-control. The next three chapters will guide you on being aware of principles of living to align your mind and body using several ancestral views on health.

Applying C.A.R.E.

Living within the C.A.R.E. framework is a lifestyle strategy. It is not a diet nor a step by step plan that you must follow in a set order. Healing is often not a linear process.

This strategy can help you gain confidence in your health needs without comparing it to the needs of those around you.

- C – control what you can, one day at a time
- A – add foods and avoid non-foods based on your ancestral biology
- R – relationships to self, people and nature
- E – experience and experiment

— 7 —

C.A.R.E. LIFESTYLE

"A healthy person has many
goals, a sick person has one"
— Anonymous

Throughout human history, there has been a desire to extend life. Ideally, most people want to live a long and happy life. Living longer being able to easily move free from excessive pain and a good mental outlook is part of the picture everyone wants. In more recent years, the term "healthspan" has been considered more desirable than "lifespan." Lifespan refers to the length of your life, while healthspan is about the quality of time spent in good physical, mental and emotional health.

Let us be realistic though, all interventions to improve health quality take time and effort. So you might be wondering when it is best to prioritise time on these new actions for self-care. While it is never too late to feel a bit better than the day before, this approach is not like surgery or

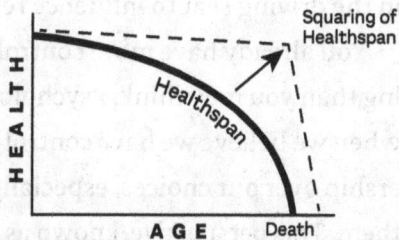

medication. All nutrition and lifestyle strategies work best when applied as soon as our optimal health declines. Implementing these strategies as soon as possible can slow this decline and even increase the chances of reversal.

A large part of your results will come down to how consistently you apply some of these strategies. It is a process that starts with taking action first, not relying on endless willpower.

The famous physicist Albert Einstein said in a letter to his son, "Life is like riding a bicycle. To keep your balance you must keep moving." I take the quotation to mean that we can get stuck or lose our way if we do not act on what we learn. We grow through learning. Learning becomes knowledge and knowledge becomes power when we choose to use it. Just as in nature, nothing alive can remain stagnant. Movement can help us get back into the flow and not be stuck.

Confidence builds from the momentum of applying new skills. Start with easy ones and have fun along the way.

C – Control What You Can

Let us start with your controllable actions. For some people, control could imply something rigid. In reality, that is not the case at all. I am not talking about forced control. I am talking about your realistic ability to affect the outcome, controls that put you in the driving seat to influence results.

You already have more control over your health and well-being than you may think. Psychology research in the 1960s found when we believe we have control or agency it helps us take ownership over our choices, especially if we know why we are doing them. This perspective, known as the "locus of control" describes the degree to which we believe certain results come from our behaviours or from forces that are external to us. Here is a daily food and lifestyle choice example.

Someone with an external locus of control might see the reason for not making enough progress on their new body size goal was that they had no spare time to grocery shop or exercise – too much spent on work or after-school kids' activities, making takeaway meals easier to organise. Someone with an internal locus of control may think they did not put enough effort into preparation to buy healthy foods to keep in the freezer or fridge for busy days. The external locus person will admit they are less inclined to have other good habits like going to bed early so they can wake up fresh for a short walk when not eating well. The internally focused person will find the power to create change.

To stay motivated I encourage you to ask yourself at any time: *What actions can I control at this moment?*

This thinking helps you start again, anytime to make better decisions and adjust them step-by-step in a way that feels good. Make little promises to yourself that you can keep, that you are confident with. This can help increase trust in yourself.

Believing in your new identity first will help you act as if you are already doing what that type of person would. View your actions based on your future self who has already achieved results. Focus on what you want, rather than reinforcing what you do not want, as it helps you stay positive and hopeful.

So what kind of small steps am I talking about?
- Create a peaceful space in your kitchen so you can focus on putting healthy ingredients on a meal.

Easy examples could include:

- Put on some calming peaceful background music.
- Wear noise-cancelling headphones if no one is talking to you and there is lots of background noise from others in the house – loud music, voices or television.

Wearing good quality headphones are one of my favourite tools to use when I want to focus and stay calm. Even without music or anything playing they can rapidly bring about a quiet, internal environment and minimise distractions.

I have seen an instant shift in calm come to those with high sensory sensitivity or anxiety from using headphones to create active silence.

Bridging The Gaps

I had never heard the saying "mind the gap" until I lived in London for a few years back in the late 90s. The gap refers to the space between the platform and the train. It is a warning sign, yet so catchy that t-shirts with this text printed can be bought everywhere in London.

Many of us, myself included, have gaps in our ability to influence results in our daily life. Let us use time as an example. How we spend our time or attention reflects our priorities. Say you want to eat better but do not make time to buy ingredients you need to make healthy meals later. Consistently putting in effort to make better choices gradually creates results. The same applies to our poorer choices. If we do not notice that *gap* between what we want and where our attention and efforts really are, we can sabotage ourselves and feel frustrated about not taking better care of ourselves. If we fall into the gap and get caught in a negative spiral of reactivity or bad habits, it can make things worse for ourselves and those around us.

What if we tried to bridge the gaps instead? If we "mind the gap", we can start to pay attention to what changes are within our control. By finding the causes that unintentionally sabotage your efforts, you can learn how to influence each gap. You may find more time, money, focus and effort available to help you make your long-term solutions stick.

Self-questioning is a great way to check in and reflect on some inner reasons you may think or feel a certain way at that moment. When did you last drink water? Or take a deep breath?

When you learn to transform habits, you will transform your life.

Habits are small decisions you make and actions you perform every day.

Researchers at Duke University found that habits account for about 40% of our behaviours on any given day. These are the things we mostly have control over too.

There are gaps between our thoughts and behaviours. Especially when it comes to addictive habits. It is the habit loop, popularized by Charles Duhigg's book, *The Power of Habit* and James Clear's book, *Atomic Habits*:

Cue – Craving – Response – Reward

The gap is the part between craving and response. It is an opportunity for awareness and attention to use different self-care activities, tools and principles, to make better choices.

One common habit we might experience is grocery shopping while hungry which might look as follows.

Walk through the snack aisle in the supermarket (cue), and your mouth begins to water when seeing chocolates and potato chips (craving). Without a pause or much consideration, you are likely to give in to the craving and the next thing, that chocolate or bag of chips ends up in your shopping basket (response), ready to unwrap and eat as soon as you leave the shop (reward).

Realising you have a typical habit response at the moment you have cravings allows you to pause and think about your response. This helps override your primitive brain and make a more conscious decision. In this case that would be to leave the chocolate bar where it is. You may worry you then miss out on a reward, but you do not! The reward is just different: It can be the feeling of proudness of your inner strength or the fact that you feel good that day as you have made healthy food choices.

Understanding how to build new habits and how current habits impact on you is essential for making progress in your health, happiness and life.

A – Add in Real Foods

Ancestral Food Foundations

This framework takes into consideration foods that were part of many thousands of years of ancestral design. Humans have been hunter-gatherers for at least 2.5 million years. Agriculture only began about 12,000 years ago. Humans were forced to adapt to eating certain foods during times of famine, war or other challenges like transportation issues. Our genes compensated for a generation or two, until health quality declined (seen from archaeological findings of human remains).

If previous generations of relatives lived through times of limited food or starvation, certain genes still hold that imprint. For this reason it is really easy to gain weight when much of our primal DNA code is 'protecting us' from times of famine by storing fat.

Many of us are often driven to choose foods based on emotional habits or norms seen in modern society and not based or led by our biology.

So when I mention ancestral health, perhaps think much further back than just the last three generations. It is unlikely to cause harm if you understand that you are not supposed to feel hungry if eating three good main meals per day. If you are hungry, then it is a clue that something important is missing from main meals. Ideally, seek one-on-one support to personalise a better eating plan.

Meal Principles that Support Brain, Gut and Epigenetic Risks

1. Avoid skipping meals
Skipping meals can trigger relapses for ALL addictive behaviours as it may cause blood sugar swings and other hormonal imbalances. To support intestinal clean up and movement, it is best to only have three main meals per day. Avoid snacking as this supports a clean-up phase of at least four hours between meals. If you really want a satisfying fat or protein "treat" to help you feel full longer and support your body then anchor this to one of your main meals.

2. Adopt a natural eating pattern
Eating at regular meal times matters. Though some individual variations apply, depending on your sleep schedule, most of us benefit from eating during daylight hours. This could mean your first meal might be within two hours of waking and last bite of

food about three hours before bed. A natural overnight fasting window of a least 12 hours daily, for example between 7am and 7pm, is ideal for most. This fits in line with ancient Ayurvedic wisdom that emphasises our "digestive fire" or strongest ability to breakdown food matches the daylight rhythm, when the sun peaks roughly between 10am and 2pm. For this reason it is especially important not to skip a main meal during this time. Establishing a routine eating pattern that aligns with rhythms of nature will stabilise hormones and brain chemicals, so your new healthy habits stick.

3. Choose nutrient-dense foods

It is ideal to aim to eat plenty of organic vegetables and some fruit but if this is unavailable or unaffordable then look for the "Clean 15" and "Dirty Dozen" list on EWG.org. Each year this non-profit organisation tests pesticide levels of conventional fruits and vegetables.

When the majority of the foods you buy and eat are whole, fresh or frozen local produce, you will naturally receive many essential nutrients. The best nutrient-dense foods to add more often include: naturally found fats, ethically sourced proteins and an abundance of vegetables, as they consistently support blood sugar and brain chemistry. This specific way of eating is a lifestyle rather than a diet. Further details for living this low-carb, healthy high-fat lifestyle, often referred to as the LCHF eating style, are detailed in the next chapter.

Many available products easily trigger addictive patterns. These include packaged meals, ultra-processed foods, sugars, unnatural fats, as well as alcohol, tobacco or hard drugs.

4. Be a good ingredients "detective"

If you regularly buy pre-packaged food or takeaway meals it is important to read product labels well. Many products in grocery stores or even health food shops have crafty marketing on the packaging that veils potentially harmful ingredients. It is easy to find a new product and overlook details of ingredients, such as additives, flavour enhancers, unnatural fats including vegetable oils and many and varied names for sugar. Keep an eye out for any pre-packaged meat or fish dishes, frozen meals, dips, sauces and many snack foods that contain these. Choose mostly unprocessed foods that do not have an ingredient list, as is the case with vegetables.

Health-suggestive words such as "natural", "fat-free", "gluten-free" or "no added sugar" on packaging can distract us. None of these terms mean certain foods are healthy though. Carefully checking the ingredients list on the back of a product is the best way to be a good detective.

It is wise to remember the saying "buyer beware", from the ancient Latin phrase caveat emptor, meaning you cannot believe everything marketing labels claim. Food processing in Australia is very similar to the USA, and new research from 2023 has determined that 60 per cent of foods purchased by Americans contain technical food additives including colouring or flavouring agents, preservatives and sweeteners.

Rather than relying on marketing spin, we have to use our own critical judgment and knowledge about time-tested principles of health and what good nutrition is when deciding what to buy for ourselves or loved ones. If the meal has a higher proportion of sugar and flour (in any form) than fat or protein, that meal is likely to spike blood sugar levels – i.e. quickly lift energy with a downward effect not long afterwards because, as discussed in Part 2, "hungry cells" lead to more cravings.

5. Use safe cookware

Eating mostly cooked, seasonal foods with a minimal amount of raw, cold foods makes digestion easier. Though it is wise to minimise eating cooked foods from plastic containers, and especially avoid reheating them. Avoid using BPA and Teflon non-stick cookware.

When you do eat, sit down, breath slowly and chew your food well, to further aid nutrient breakdown and improve absorption. Remember from Chapter 4 that enzymes from our saliva and pancreas, along with our stomach acid (hydrochloric acid) are foundations of good digestion. Eating slowly and while calm is a good lifelong practice to adopt.

R – for Relationships With Yourself and Others

Back in my early career as a flight attendant, I would do the safety demonstration before take-off. You are probably familiar with the part that says, "Fit your own mask first before assisting others". This is a relevant part of our life, as we really cannot give much to others without looking after ourselves.

All sorts of triggers overwhelm us when we lack self-care. It is easy to fall back on old habits using harmful substances to numb uncomfortable feelings of being overwhelmed or burnt out unless we have a nourishing plan.

You might want to tell yourself that you do not have time for self-care. The reality though is the more stressed you are and the less time you have to do it, the more you need to do it. As a matter of fact, you are likely to be overwhelmed by busyness *because* you are not doing enough of the right self-care, not the other way around. The more stressed you are the more self-care you need.

Skipping meals, living on less sleep, not getting time outside daily or feeling like you have to do it all and do it all "perfectly" only depletes you further. I encourage you to create some space to prioritise self-care. Make it an essential part of a lifelong lifestyle. Even if you currently are not doing well with it, it is a learnable skill that you can get good at. One I am sure you will want to try if you have taken time out to read this book.

When practising basic self-care, you become more efficient at prioritising things, removing unessential chores and getting resourceful by finding support or professional help.

What are these basics of self-care? Here is a list to get you started:

- fill your fridge with real whole foods including proteins, fats and vegetables
- stay adequately hydrated
- move your body every day even by walking or dancing around the house to some fun music
- spend regular time in nature, even if it's just the local park
- take a soothing bath with Epsom salts
- ask for, seek (or hire) help

This is just the beginning.

When in parasympathetic (rest and digest) mode more often, anything that throws you out of it feels so uncomfortable. You will want to reset back as soon as you can. Once new memories are formed in your brain, new feelings or sensations will give you confidence to continue. We only know what we know!

Unfortunately, many people do not know what it feels like to be really well, until they do.

It is about living in a mode of self-compassion, staying positive and hopeful about what you can control. In essence, you are likely stressed and running around because you are not prioritising the right self-care habits yet. Here is a chance to start.

Six Powerful Self-Care Pillars

1. Sleep Quality

In the body the lymphatic vessels are pathways for our tissue to flush out circulating waste, excess fluid and toxins through our kidneys, bowels and sweat from the skin. For a long time, scientists thought the brain did not detoxify. That is, until 2013 when a new discovery was made. This revealed our brains have a similar waste system called the glymphatic system. This system controls the flow of cerebrospinal fluid and keeps metabolic waste and toxins from accumulating around brain cells.

While we sleep our brain cells shrink and this creates a 60 percent increase in interstitial space around neurons, which means more efficient glymphatic flow to detoxify our brain. When we do not sleep well, we do not cleanse our brains and remove as much waste.

Optimising sleep is critical for us to reach our full potential. Here are some strategies to try:

Eat dinner early and eat enough

Ideally, before 7pm as our digestion slows when the sun sets. Eating enough blood sugar-stabilising foods like protein, fat and slow-burning carbs (such as sweet potato or pumpkin) for your body size will help avoid going to sleep hungry. If you are experiencing a very stressful period and your blood glucose is unstable during the day it may also dip during the night, which can make you wake up (nocturnal hypoglycaemia). If you regularly have a hard time staying asleep then fewer toxins are cleared from your brain, which means less than optimal repair.

Wind down slowly with some sleep prep
Play some calming background music, or wear headphones and listen to a meditation app – or just enjoy silence with your thoughts and breath to help you unwind before bed. Disconnect from digital screens one hour before bedtime to help increase melatonin, the sleep hormone. Some healthy relaxation routines recommended are deep belly breathing for a few minutes, meditation exercises, and taking a few minutes to keep a journal before bed. For others reading a positive, calming book or listening to the right audiobook helps. What you watch, listen to or do before you go to bed influences how well you sleep. Avoid stressful experiences as much as possible, such as the news, for a few hours before bedtime.

Ideally, be in bed for sleep by 10pm
Your brain loves routine. Ancient wisdom supports this by observing the patterns of nature that align with the energy of our bodies. The Ayurvedic Organ Clock can be used as a guide to understanding your energy cycle with a 24-hour cycle. It says our digestive organs, stomach and small intestine, repair around 10pm to 12pm every night. In my time as a shift worker, I know this can be very challenging if your income relies on different schedules. Return to a pattern that mirrors nature, with night and day, as much as possible on the days you can.

Try a weighted blanket

Weighted blankets mimic a healing touch. The light pressure has been shown to reduce cortisol and boost oxytocin (which is the "love hormone" that quickly helps with adrenal recovery). They are great for light sleepers, sensitive brains or those who are recovering from emotional stress. I have personally found them to be wonderful when hormone levels shift for women in their 40s, affecting sleep quality.

Try wearing a continuous glucose monitor (CGM) for 14 days to observe any low blood sugar spikes in the middle of the night that may disrupt sleep quality. Hormonal changes throughout a woman's menstrual cycle can influence blood sugar sensitivity to diets and stress tolerance. Track any low blood sugar swings after eating certain foods or emotional tension. Large surges from high to low levels can impact on mood with irritability, lack of focus and fatigue. Daily arguments or stressful relationships can increase blood sugar levels regardless of dietary choices. I was surprised when I wore a continuous glucose monitor for 14 days to check how high my own blood sugars were on stressful mornings at home without eating anything at all.

2. Breathing, Mindfulness and Meditation

To talk about optimising genes and lowering our predisposed risk towards negative behaviours or disease would be incomplete without discussion. The key connection between our breath and emotions lies with changes in the speed and depth of our breathing. Whatever emotion we experience, be it sadness, anger, joy or fear, each has a corresponding rhythm of the breath.

Have you ever noticed how you breathe when you are angry

or feel overwhelmed? Uncontrolled stress activates your sympathetic nervous system, which might cause you to hold your breath, breathe faster or more shallowly. This reduces oxygen circulating in our body and makes it hard to think and prepare to "fight or flight."

Depending on the intensity of the situation, our breath will rarely be slow, relaxed or deep. When we activate calm, rhythmic, deep breathing, we relax the nervous system into a more dominant "rest and digest" mode – sending a signal of safety to our mind and body.

A really simple way to reset and soothe those fried nerves starts with tuning in to how you breathe. Once you have focused on your breath, inhale through your nose, with your mouth closed, and slowly breathe down deep into your belly. Calming your breath expands your perspective, allowing you to think more clearly and with control over your next choices. Breathing well gets you closer to maximum energy and vitality.

The technical reasons behind this are fascinating. As James Nestor explains: "Breathing slow, less and through the nose balances levels of respiratory gases in the body and sends the maximum amount of oxygen to the maximum amount of tissues so that our cells have the maximum amount of electron reactivity."

It is no wonder many Eastern medical systems place a core emphasis on aligning mind and body through breath. Ayurveda calls it Pranayama. The Chinese call their system of conscious breathing exercises Qigong: Qi, meaning "energy (breath being one form)," and gong, meaning work, exercise or achievement. Higher-level qigong practices such as Falun Gong refer to "gong" as "cultivation energy." According to both Ayurveda and traditional Chinese medicine, breath work expands our life force.

Five years before my first experience of the Falun Gong exercises I was a regular yoga devotee. Body stretching movements in yoga and aligning focus of the mind and breath were good starting points for me in the Eastern healing arts. However, maintaining that calm energy outside of yoga classes did not come with ease. When I switched to practicing qigong and incorporating mediation, I found a deeper state of peace with lasting effects.

Qigong is a traditional Chinese movement practice for promoting health that includes slow movements, breathing exercises and meditation. Beneficial health effects are found in a vast amount of research on qigong, meditation and specifically Falun Gong.

Meditation Study Highlights

◆ A 2000 to 2015 longitudinal cohort study of terminal cancer patients in China showed remarkable results on the effectiveness of meditation and mind-body practice – specifically the practice of Falun Gong. The study focused on 152 patients who had terminal cancer, all of whom practised Falun Gong. 149 (98%) of them were still alive in 2016. Among those still alive, 65 patients experienced cancer treatment failure, 74 did not take any further cancer treatment after diagnosis, and 13 received treatment alongside the Falun Gong practice.

◆ In 2020, researchers from the Psychology Department of the University of California measured hemispheric brain changes using a brain attention test called ELANT. The study researchers focused on brain regions corresponding to emotion and conflict resolution. They demonstrated that 19 long-term practitioners of Falun Gong had higher hemispheric activity levels compared to 16 controls after 91 minutes of qigong exercise. The changes were deemed positive as the more active brain regions in the long-term practitioners related to conflict resolution and positive emotions.

◆ A 2020 publication in the Journal of Psychosomatic Medicine by Dr. Margaret Trey recommended the usefulness of Falun Gong in working with clients experiencing traumatic stress due to its ability to alleviate anxiety and bring inner peace.

◆ Research on various other forms of meditation and mind–body interventions, between 2012 and 2018 demonstrated reduced gene expression of genes that can lead to inflammation. A 2017 meta-analysis, reviewing eight studies on meditation and physiological markers of stress, found reduced blood pressure and cortisol levels.

A term that has dramatically risen in mainstream popularity during the past 15 years is mindfulness. Mindfulness is the skill or practice that one builds while meditating. Having conscious awareness of your thoughts, feelings, and the sensations around you is a practice you can take with you throughout any day. Although mindfulness stems from ancient Buddhist philosophy, it has become part of wellness programs of numerous corporate businesses worldwide.

Gradually learning to calm painful emotions, stop constant thoughts or worries about the future and feel emotional acceptance is a large part of mindfulness. Modern research studies (2005 and 2012) even validate how entwined our spirituality, life experience, and physical bodies are.

Both mindfulness and meditation can help one focus, with greater awareness, on the present moment. At whatever starting point you are at, these practices encourage inner calm.

3. Vagus Nerve Stimulation

Vagus nerve stimulation involves altering activation of the parasympathetic nervous system's main component that connects many different organs with your brain. These interventions can turn down the "fight and flight" sympathetic mode that may be triggered by withdrawing a substance or other habits it can bring about. Vagus nerve stimulation allows us to think more clearly in a relaxed, calm state which helps us make rational healthy choices. Here are two simple interventions that stimulate the vagus nerve.

Here are two simple interventions that stimulate the vagus nerve.

- **Physiological sigh**
  Stanford researchers discovered an easy breathing pattern, called a physiological sigh, can temporarily stimulate the vagus nerve. This breathing pattern involves two inhales through the nose, followed by an extended exhale through the mouth.

- **Cold water therapy**
  Very cold water causes an abrupt sensory change that stimulates the vagus nerve, which causes our heart and breathing rate to slow down, shifting us into a calmer and more parasympathetic state.

Remarkable increases in dopamine levels have been measured from being submerged in water at 14 degrees Celsius (57F). A huge 250 per cent boost of dopamine could be seen in participants from this small cold water therapy study.

The first time I experienced an ice bath submersion in an 8-degree Celsius (46F) plunge bath, I felt every level of my nervous system. First, intense shock – full "fight and flight" mode – wanting to get out within seconds, with determination and encouragement I resisted that urge, slowed my breathing, and stayed in long enough to relax. Supportive staff at the venue I was at guided and encouraged me from 2.5 minutes the first time, to over seven minutes on the fourth day. This made a world of difference in distracting me from looking at the timer or focusing on cold sensations. Even though I was tempted to rush straight to a hot shower when I first exited, I took their advice and warmed up naturally. In about half an hour I had a hot shower and afterwards felt extremely alert, refreshed and energised. My sleep improved dramatically that night and a few after that short trial. It may be something you would like to experience to see how you respond.

4. Gratitude For Wellbeing
Some qigong and meditation practices further enhance physical benefits by opening a space to feel gratitude in the body. Gratitude can soothe our nervous system. In the brain gratitude activates the

hypothalamus with the rest of the limbic system, which regulates emotions and keeps us in balance (homeostasis).

The science has been around for decades. Numerous studies of consistent gratitude practices have shown an increase in long-term happiness and our ability to cope with stressful events. Having a grateful disposition can reduce the risk of burnout, symptoms of depression and materialism. It generally makes you happier and brings about emotional balance. For thousands of years gratitude was passed on from one generation to another in traditional cultures. Immediately, accessing gratitude in a moment can make you feel more at ease and content.

There are many methods you can use to introduce more thankfulness into your life.

Gratitude journals are known to be particularly good for many, but do you keep one? I too struggled with trying to keep a gratitude journal. When I most needed to find positivity in my life, making a gratitude list was just not a habit I could stick with. It felt like it was something I had to force myself to do.

I instinctively knew what it was like to "feel gratitude" in my body. This is when we embody emotions and experience the benefits of gratitude – which is another part of that mind–body connection mentioned in previous chapters. When every cell of our body feels "thankful" or sees someone mirror this message to us, it sends a signal of psychological safety to our mind as well.

Many years after learning the calming qigong exercises of Falun Gong, I had a revelation. I noticed in the music instructions I heard one word more frequently throughout the first exercise. The hand movements follow the music, and the word Heshi was said not just once but 24 times. In Chinese, Heshi means, "press the hands together" and is a gesture used when someone wants to express deeply sincere gratitude. This gesture, Heshi, can also represent "please" and "I'm sorry", and even has spiritual associations. Throughout this nine-minute qigong exercise my body felt and expressed gratitude without any mental effort. No wonder I felt more relaxed and happier afterwards.

In the West there is not much reverence given to this gesture, though in recent years a new folded hands emoji symbol has been included on smartphones. You may be familiar with this traditional gesture from yoga. It is often used by people living in South Asia, still very common today in Thailand, where the majority are Buddhists. It is a daily greeting, used when praying, showing respect to a spiritual teacher or when facing the image of a divine being.

Those times when you are overwhelmed or feeling unappreciated it is easy to think there is not enough of anything. "Not enough, time, money, health, support," and the list continues. Gratitude can help you have more positive feelings and less negative ones. It can create a wedge of hope. When you build on that daily, bit by bit your state can widen to see the bigger picture outside those hard days and shift out of survival mode.

When you are naturally in a state of abundance, you might notice more contentment and space for yourself and some left to give to others. Maybe share kindness with a smile or choose a healthy bite to eat instead of a harmful trigger.

Recent research by Dr Emiliana Simon-Thomas, science director at the Greater Good Science Center, linked gratitude with changes in our physiology, reduced blood pressure and strengthened tone of the vagus nerve for a relaxed and parasympathetic state.

If you tend to overthink things or prefer a more kinaesthetic, physical body, experience, perhaps try some form of movement to embody gratitude. A simple self-hug is easy. Feel appreciation in your body to create some positivity if consistently writing a journal is not your thing. Fill yourself with gratitude and goodness, in whatever form you choose to feel empowered in the present moment.

5. Movement for Mood
Advice from the high-performance coaching world says:
mood follows action

Take this example:
- Can you remember a morning you woke up and really did not want to get out of bed? Maybe you lay there, thinking of all the reasons not to move.
- Did you feel worse the longer you lay there?
- Did you feel more stuck?

Action can shift your state of mind and mood by moving your body. If you get out of bed, have a shower then go for a walk in the fresh air your body usually starts to feel better. Our behaviours bring our moods along with them.

Moving my body, even a little, works wonders for me. It can stop me from overthinking things. Any type of body movement can bring a lighter and brighter perspective into my day. The right kind of moving or stretching can also be a natural way to feel more awake and alert throughout the day.

Listening to music or a podcast while walking the nearby hills, doing weights or a cycle class at the gym, weeding my garden, qigong and dancing in my living room to some upbeat tunes with my son are my favourite ways to move. When I lived near the ocean or visited a local pool to enter the water, even floating as if I were weightless, this brought instant relief. The best actions are those that take almost no effort to start and have other benefits go along with it. Maybe seeing a friend as you walk to the coffee shop or at your local gym. Once this happy memory is stored, it is easy to repeat. The right kind of movement should give you energy and lift your mood. Give it a try next time you feel stuck.

An easy motto to remember: *Move to change your mood*.

Another phrase that can be a great action reset, if you notice you lose your calm, get frazzled or upset is: *Stop, drop and roll*.

- *stop* what you are doing
- calm down and *drop* into your body; notice your breathing
- then *roll* on with what you were doing.

The science of why our movement affects our mood is again related to chemical changes in our brains. Neurotransmitters stimulate neurons in our brain to take action. Hormones stimulate cells outside your brain into action.

You may have heard of adrenaline also called epinephrine. Like dopamine, it is both a hormone and neurotransmitter that stimulates action. Epinephrine stimulates our energy and alertness. Many of the lifestyle and food recommendations in this book improve the levels and function of all neurotransmitters.

If you want more energy, take small actions you may doubt you have energy for. This can boost epinephrine, as humans need to *move more and breathe more*.

That means increasing energy levels is not possible through physically sitting down all day. The easiest places to start are:

- Moderate/intense exercise at least three times a week for 20 minutes – cycling, jogging or hill walking with a bit of intensity to move beyond the comfort zone.
- Nature-based movement like hiking or swimming offers even better health benefits.
- Qigong, previously discussed for its other benefits, has slow-moving exercises that may look easy yet are very challenging and mood-enhancing to perform.

Doing these movements outdoors, weather permitting, can bring many extra benefits. A recent meta-analysis of 50 studies examined nature-based outdoor activities for mental and physical health and found that gardening, green exercise plus nature-based therapy all improve mental health outcomes in adults – including those with pre-existing mental health problems.

When we reconnect with nature and ground ourselves in mind and body we support our nervous system to rebalance and thus regain control over our health potential.

6. Strengthening Your Emotional Health

Balancing your emotions comes more naturally when your nervous system is calm and your physical body has its necessities taken care of. Take one step at a time. Day by day.

Words we say to ourselves have power. When the time is right for your healing stage, finding words to express any deeply buried emotions can bring about new perspectives. No one other than you has to see or hear those words to benefit. Finding a personal narrative in words to explain our thoughts and experiences can help unravel patterns of disorganised thinking and reduce a tendency to have those feelings remain stored in our bodies (implode) – or hurt others by releasing them (explode).

According to Mathew Lieberman, psychology professor at the University of California LA, when we give language to our experience and put something in words we move blood flow to the prefrontal cortex (brain centre for emotion regulation and perspective), away from our amygdala (our impulsive, fear centre). Lieberman and colleagues conducted MRI testing in a study in 2007 where participants had significantly diminished emotional reactivity in the amygdala region of their brains when they used words to label feelings.

Excessive emotional stress harms our genes and all cell functions. Becoming aware of your triggers and knowing how to express emotions can be part of preventing self-sabotage as you take new actions to heal. Create plans for other daily non-food rewards ahead of time such as travelling, working out, going for a drive, a walk or reconnecting with an old friend to help you quickly shift from a low emotional state.

Incorporate *peaceful pauses* into your day with these simple resets:
- stop for a minute and take in three deep breaths
- look up into the far corner of the room you are in, or even better, look out the window at the sky, clouds or nature
- go outside for at least five minutes for some fresh air and pay attention to the colour of trees, birds or butterflies flying by

- hug yourself by holding or gently stroking both sides of your arms (a technique called havening).

Incorporating saunas and cold-water plunge baths into weekly well-being strategies is also worthwhile. Physical and mental benefits include muscle recovery, relaxation, stress reduction and detoxification. For traditional hot rock saunas, start with a 15-minute session and build up over time to a maximum of 20- to 30 minutes each week. For most healthy people, infrared saunas can usually be sustained for a longer duration than traditional hot rock saunas. They feel less hot and there is hardly any significant difference shown in the benefits of using either sauna type.

These lifestyle tools will strengthen your mind and allow you will gradually create new behaviours.This will help calm hyper-sensitive nervous systems and lower stress hormones.

Better behavioural patterns can mean:
- You'll recover quicker if triggered, and still be able to stay present and connected with others
- You'll learn to trust yourself and others again.
- You'll make better decisions about how to approach challenges in life and be a more confident, better version of yourself.

Social Belonging
As humans, we all have a biological need to belong and feel cared for.

To be excluded from a community in the old days would mean risking survival. No matter how ideal our genes or eating and exercise habits are, the social aspect of health cannot be overlooked.

The negative health effects of loneliness have become the forefront of research in recent years.

Lonely people are more likely to have depression, low immunity, poor sleep, addiction risks and a shorter lifespan. Also if you have ever socially withdrawn or disconnected for long periods, you may already know it can feel awkward when in a large social situation again. Our brains can become even more hyperalert, negative or distrustful.

Even more importantly in our digital age of online interactions, the quality and reliability of our social connections matter most, not the quantity. Surrounding yourself with others who have the qualities that you want to develop is important. Dr David McClelland, a social psychologist at Harvard, found people we habitually associate with can determine as much as 95 per cent of our success or failure in life. While I prefer to think that success looks different to each of us and is not determined by one factor alone, there is no doubt that social belonging matters to all of us.

Research supports social connection as a powerful intervention for addiction recovery. A fascinating study on rats by American psychologist Dr. Bruce Alexander demonstrated an interesting comparison of addictive behaviours seen in those isolated or those belonging to a group. Dr Alexander observed that when rats were placed alone in a cage with a bottle of regular water and a bottle of cocaine-infused water, they drank the cocaine-infused water to the point of illness and death.

However, when the rats had some companions (other rats) and things to play on – toys and wheels – they drank the regular water and avoided the cocaine water. Dr Alexander's study correlates with human studies that show the importance of human belonging.

Positive Loving Connections

Belgian psychotherapist and popular author Ester Perel says the "quality of our relationships determines the quality of our lives". This is a statement the healthiest- and oldest- living people in the world would agree with too. The Okinawan people of Japan are renowned for their longevity and emphasis on a close community-oriented mindset. They are put into small groups from a young age, which acts as a safety net for companionship, and emotional and financial support.

When you know that someone deeply cares about you and that your existence in this world matters, it can pull you through the hardest of times. I have witnessed this in some of my own family, whose genes have set them up for health challenges.

My maternal grandparents are a living testament to the power of loving connection to buffer remarkable health risks. They have been married for more than 52 years, the second time around for them both. At the time of writing this book, they still live independently in their own home! Despite their many physical ailments and growing up with far less exposure to dietary pesticides, additives or environmental pollutants than in our modern world, their deep connection gave them a degree of resilience. No doubt their loving bond and simple, independent way of living has had a major role in their longevity.

Brain messages and neurochemicals have wide-reaching influence and benefits in the body. Oxytocin is a neurochemical, a brain hormone, that helps humans bond and has numerous benefits for our social attachment. It is released after childbirth, breastfeeding and deep intimacy with trust and romantic love. It influences human relations by activating the brain's reward system (via dopamine release) and regulating the parasympathetic nervous system. In other words, it acts like a drug, lowering anxiety and pain. The science about these hormones is there to verify what humans have instinctively known to be crucial for reaching the maximum longevity potential of a species. They are safe, caring connections that enhance our quality of life.

Avoid Harmful Connections

Surrounding yourself with supportive people, even if their views are not the same as yours, can positively impact your health. The opposite is also true and creates a downward spiral of harm.

Regular exposure to negative criticism, harsh verbal tones or other abuse can take a serious toll on our whole health.

We can usually choose our friends. Family is another story.

Kelly was one of my dear patients who went through years of harsh negative emotions at home whenever her teenage step-daughter came to visit. Being diagnosed with a serious chronic disease shortly before I met Kelly made her take on some major improvements to her self-care. Kelly knew she needed to nurture her emotional health for her physical body to survive.

Skills for emotional health were absent from the standard education most of us received. However, the basic emotional needs we seek to feel from those around us lie in our instincts.

The main aspects you likely want to feel are:

- safety – psychological and physical in your environment
- you can express your boundaries – stating what you need to feel safe using "I feel, I want" etc.
- sense of care – belonging with others in your environment.

In addition to food and lifestyle changes, Kelly spoke up more often and honestly about her need to feel calm most of the time at home, especially during meals, to recover and be well again. By asking for help from her husband and stepdaughter, starting first with mealtimes, she expressed a boundary without assuming others knew that she felt like she was walking on eggshells beforehand. It took assumptions away and did not come across as an attack or criticism. Thankfully Kelly is in remission and this experience has positively influenced the health of the rest of her family too.

Negative emotions are difficult to deflect due to the mirror neurons in our brains, as discussed in Chapter 5. As a reminder, these neurons enable us to mirror emotions we see in others, which helps us connect intimately. Being with someone who is angry or anxious will also affect your emotional state. Developing skills that embody emotional calm and staying compassionate will make it easier to peacefully deal with those intense emotions we all face sometimes.

E – for Experimentation

Personalise your food choices and lifestyle activities from where you are most eager to experiment first. Rarely will people change everything at once.

Perhaps start with trying one new main meal and one new vegetable you want to increase eating and make delicious for its health benefits. Build on improvements gradually while being sure to enjoy the process of learning these skills.

Here is what your "next best" choice might look like: Replace a bowl of pasta with roasted vegetables and protein, like grilled salmon or chicken, for a week.

Another option might be replacing a wheat-based cereal with

100 percent organic oats, which will lessen your intake of environmental toxins like pesticides or additives that are often added to standard cereals.

There is always a better swap option and the choice is yours. The framework of food and lifestyle choices from C.A.R.E. is offered as a guide that you fill out, based on your timeline and circumstances. We become more resilient through experimentation. The easiest way to do this is to understand flexibility and adaptability of mind. This can help strengthen our ability to thrive in new environments which embodies resilience.

For any organism, resilience comes from having a little stress and becoming stronger from it, just like how muscle grows from the pressure of lifting heavy weights. Interestingly, part of why organic plant food is believed to be better for our health than non-organic is the understanding that resilience in any organism comes from having some level of helpful stress. When a plant is partially stressed by its environment and is not shielded from insects and disease by pesticides and herbicides, it has to generate inner robustness to build immunity. A few natural environmental stressors pass on some benefits of better resilience.

When We Understand Our Role, We Have Some Control

If you keep an open, experimental mind while learning skills to nourish yourself it makes the experience more fun and gives you the power to stay in control. It helps you know what suits you best.

Hold onto this mindset if some food and recipe ideas are exploring new territory for you.

The good news is we are never neutral with our health. Regardless of your history it never too late to start. Every new and positive effort adds up. We spiral upward or downward with our health – for better or worse in one way or another. Your actions will change the direction.

Food is powerful information for your mind and body to rebalance. When you regularly add more nutrient-rich and plant-rich foods, the changes will accumulate similar to a landscaping renovation in your garden.

Imagine the "weeds" (i.e. bad bacteria, fungus and parasites), will not have as much space to grow when new plants (i.e. good bacteria) are "fertilised" with helpful foods to grow stronger and flourish. This shift takes time, personal experience and an awareness that what you currently crave *will* change once you feed your gut bacteria with different fuel.

— 8 —

EAT, DRINK AND SUPPLEMENT WITH C.A.R.E.

"Without proper nutrition, medicine is of little use... with proper nutrition, medicine is of little need."
— Charaka Samhita

Your body responds to everything you put in your mouth by influencing health risks. Your genes determine the effects of this influence through the presence of, or lack of, nutrients in your body. There is no 'neutral' effect of food or nutrition.

How well and how many ultra-processed foods or sugars versus real, whole foods you can handle is unique to you. All nutritional inputs accumulate, either leading to nutrient imbalances or optimal health.

To help you live with C.A.R.E., in this chapter, we will dive deeper into the foods to *add* and those to avoid.

Realistically, six to 12 weeks is recommended for these suggestions to have a lasting effect. However, some people experience huge changes within as little as four weeks. Pace yourself by taking one day at a time when focusing on better food choices. Remember though, food and lifestyle approaches take time and persistence.

Including more nourishing, additive-free and unprocessed foods daily will safely fast-track your results. Take heart that if you are not ready to change your current eating style then you can still benefit from the other lifestyle practices in the plan. You make it work for you, applying what you want, when you are ready.

The following strategies are beneficial for most people with genetically sensitive brains or who have addictive tendencies. The benefits also extend to those who have been stuck with unresolved chronic stress or have been struggling with sleep and focus issues. The common theme here is to provide nervous system support, which is central to brain health.

These guidelines are for addressing dysfunctional brain patterns. Remember from Chapter 4, we have nine times more nerve signals coming from our gut (intestines) to our brain than signals from our brain to our gut. What we eat or do not eat daily directly affects our brain and thus our behaviour, mood and outlook in life.

Macro Matters

Macronutrients are substances our body needs in large amounts to provide energy and fuel all bodily functions. You have likely heard of the main three macronutrients: Proteins, fats and carbohydrates.

To explain their roles:
- Protein is for tissue growth and DNA repair
- Fat is for hormones, cell membranes, promoting fullness and slow-burning energy
- Carbohydrates are for fast-burning energy

Let us dig a little bit deeper.

Protein

Protein stems from the Greek word *proteois* for "primary," meaning "in the lead" or "standing in front." Adequate daily protein is extremely important for proper growth and maintenance of the human body, at every life stage.

Protein is broken down into amino acids which are used by our cells. These are essential for repairing all tissues including damaged DNA. What is often overlooked is that amino acids feed your brain chemicals (neurotransmitters) that make you feel happy, calm, motivated, able to sleep when you need and feel good overall. Protein helps keep your blood sugar level balanced, is also used in hormone and enzyme production, helps your immune system fight infections and can be used as a backup energy source if needed.

Adequate intake is one of the most important things to focus on in any time of mental or physical recovery. It keeps cognitive thought processes working well, which gives good judgment – a vital tool to help stay rational or avoid addictive habits.

Foods high in unprocessed protein include grass-fed or organic red meat, wild kangaroo fillets, poultry, wild-caught fatty fish, seafood, free-range eggs and organic dairy products. It is important to read the ingredients list of all packaged meat or fish. For those following a plant-based diet, non-GMO soy products like tempeh or tofu and legumes are good sources of protein. Many vegetarian protein substitutes are highly processed with new synthetic ingredients that are not recognised by our cells or supportive of good health.

How Much Protein Do You Need?

The amount of protein you need is based on your body weight

and age. The general rule for adults is one gram of protein per 1 kilogram of ideal body weight. More is required if you are more than moderately physically active. If you weigh 60kg that does not mean your body can break down 60 grams of protein in one meal. Generally, 20 to 30 grams of protein at each meal is best. When split over two or three meals per day, this is a realistic way for your body to break it down and is achievable for most people.

Busy people, who are used to breakfast cereal sometimes find it hard to include protein at this time. I often recommend one scoop of grass-fed or organic whey protein. Whey has a high and fast rate of absorption. It is a rich source of leucine for muscle growth and cysteine, which is a crucial amino acid for glutathione synthesis (a major antioxidant).

Fats

Dietary fat breaks down into fatty acids that are vital for brain functions, cell membranes and vitamin absorption. Fat makes us feel full for longer, is the backbone of our hormones and influences inflammatory processes.

To keep it simple, the fats we often eat fit into two categories – natural and unnatural. Healthy fats are natural fats with few ingredients and found closest to their original form: Extra virgin oil, avocado, ghee, coconut oil and 100% butter. Unnatural fats are found in most processed foods as various forms of vegetable oil or seed oils (such as canola oil) and sold as cooking oil sprays and margarine (called vegetable spreads, often blended with real butter to make them sound natural). Most vegetable and seed oils require a high degree of processing to last longer on the supermarket shelf and are not naturally in liquid form at room temperature.

The term "essential fatty acids" refers to fats commonly known as Omega 3 and Omega 6. These are both polyunsaturated types of fat that we need to consume daily, as our body cannot make them on its own. It is crucial to get the balance of these fatty acids right to keep their different functions in check, including our body's inflammation load. Studies have shown that the optimal level of omega-3 to 6 ratios is about 4:1. Eating a typical Western diet a person consumes a ratio of 15:1 Omega-6 to Omega-3. Omega 6 fats, found in ultra-processed foods, are cheaper to buy and easily damaged or oxidised when heated at high temperatures. An accumulation of oxidised Omega 6 fats damages DNA and promotes high inflammation levels.

Most dips, sauces, chips, snack bars, and most takeaway foods contain vegetable oils high in Omega 6. Vegetable oils made with corn, soy and canola are often genetically modified, which causes further harm.

Carbohydrates

When eating carbohydrates (carbs), your body breaks them down into simple sugar molecules, mainly glucose. These sugar molecules enter your bloodstream and serve as energy for cells.

Not all carbs are equal in the way our body handles them. Until the processed food industry entered our world, carbs used to fit into two broad categories – simple and complex (which includes fibre). Refined carbohydrates are a newer term you may have heard of. Refined carbs are those that have had their nutrients removed during processing, making them simple carbs, even if they were once from a complex source. One example of this is a sweet potato (complex) made into sweet potato chips (simple).

Simple carbs are usually for fast-acting energy and have a high glycaemic (GI) effect, that quickly enters your bloodstream and raises your blood sugar level and is then either used up by the cells or stored as fat. High GI examples are fruit juices, sugars (especially fructose), soft drinks and candy that provide little or no nutritional value. High GI foods require a higher amount of insulin (a fat-storage hormone) to be released to allow glucose to enter cells.

Refined carbs are similar to simple carbs but additional processing has removed any fibre, vitamins and minerals that the food may have contained. Because of this, refined carbs rapidly increase blood sugar and insulin levels. Examples of refined carbs include bread, pasta and white rice. If refined carbs are a regular feature in the diet, they have been shown to gradually cause all sorts of inflammation and hormone problems. I often hear patients say, "*I have removed sugars from my diet*" and then find out they are having a couple of servings of fruit per day, sandwiches for lunch and a bowl of pasta for dinner. Not only is this diet high in simple carbohydrates (which are types of sugars) but also low in protein, which, as we have discussed, is a vital essential macronutrient deficiency to address first.

Complex carbs contain longer chains of sugar molecules (polysaccharides), which take longer to enter the bloodstream. Complex carbs are found in wholegrains and legumes and are also abundant in root vegetables like carrot, pumpkin and beetroot. The healthiest carbohydrates come from plant foods with fibre still intact. Fibre is the non-digestible part of the carbohydrate. There are three types of fibre, so it is important to have a combination of them for full benefits as they can make you feel full. The three types are: Soluble, insoluble and resistant starch. Soluble fibres dissolve in water and slow down your digestion and bowels.

Examples of foods containing soluble fibre are most legumes, psyllium and wholegrains like barley. Insoluble fibres feed your gut microbiome, soften the contents of the bowels and speed up the emptying process. Examples of foods containing soluble fibre are most legumes, psyllium and wholegrains like barley. Insoluble types of fibre feed your gut microbiome, soften the contents of the bowels and speed up the emptying process. Examples are cabbage, broccoli, most dark green leafy veggies and unpeeled fruits, especially pears, all of which help relieve constipation. Resistant starches are not absorbed yet provide fuel for good bacteria in our large intestine while protecting the bowel lining. Resistant starch has also been shown to lower the severity of insulin resistance. Examples of resistant starches are oats, cooked then cooled potatoes, and green or under-ripe bananas.

Nature's best forms of carbohydrates are plant-rich sources of vegetables containing folate, which provides even broader benefits. As I discussed in Chapter 4, regularly eating adequate folate-rich foods is important if you have MTHFR gene variations.

The following table may help prioritise your plant-rich carbohydrate choices.

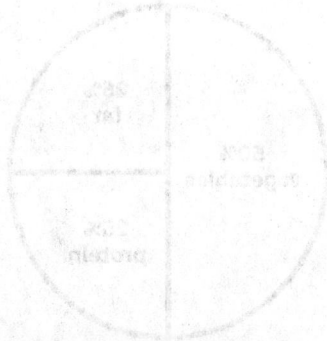

Folate – Containing Foods	Micrograms (mcg) DFE per serving
Lentils, cooked, 1/2 cup	180
Arugula (rocket), raw 100gm	97
Rice, white, cooked, 1/2 cup†	90 (avoid if added synthetic folic acid)
Asparagus, boiled, 4 spears	89
Brussels sprouts, frozen, boiled, 1/2 cup	78
Kale, lightly cooked, 1 cup	65
Lettuce, romaine, shredded, 1 cup	64
Avocado, raw, sliced, 1/2 cup	59
Broccoli, chopped, frozen, cooked, 1/2 cup	52
Mustard greens, chopped, boiled, 1/2 cup	52
Green peas, frozen, boiled, 1/2 cup	47
Kidney beans, canned, 1/2 cup	46

While carbohydrates provide energy, fuel for gut bacteria and other benefits to the digestive tract from fibre, your cells require much more than just energy to function well. Protein and fat have many more vital functions for our hormones and various pathways throughout our whole body. Adequate protein, fat and fibre based on your current age and body size, should be the foundation of healthy meals.

Here is a visual of a healthy mix of foods on a plate:

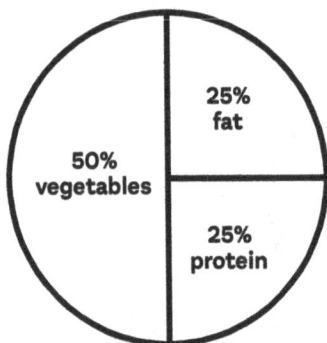

Key Bioactive Supplements

Certain molecules or nutrients are more biologically active and beneficial for the human body to thrive. These supplements can complement a healthy diet to get faster results, as they support primary gene pathways and metabolic cellular functions, promote better detoxification and reduce inflammation.

Correct 'food first' principles are more important, though, with our modern stressful lives, food alone is rarely enough to reduce inflammatory and environmental toxin loads.

Especially difficult for many is reaching sufficient Omega 3s from fatty fish and eating plenty of green leafy vegetables.

The saying "less is more" applies to how many supplements you may require. Taking too many different supplements is not the solution. Better-sourced and manufactured brands provide superior results.

Best Absorption

Brand quality and the form of supplement delivery can make a huge difference in absorption. There is an absorption ranking order that naturopaths and nutritionists use to obtain maximum results from reputable product brands. Intravenous delivery (IV) directly into blood needs medical assistance, so it is excluded from this list. Within our bodies, there is a scale from easy to hard to absorb when it comes to nutrient or herbal delivery.

That order is:

- Liquid (incl. liposomal)
- Powder (incl. capsules and chewable forms)
- Tablets

Tablets are cheaper to manufacture and you may be wasting your money. While the temptation to buy cheaper priced tablets may look appealing many retail brand tablets may have harmful binders and fillers, thus less absorption of the main important nutrients.

Seven Powerful Performers

1. Sulphoraphane (broccoli sprouts)
2. Magnesium
3. Zinc
4. L-Theanine
5. Omega 3s
6. Vitamin D
7. Spirulina

1. Sulphoraphane (Broccoli Sprouts)

Every day, as we age, our bodies are constantly protecting us by eliminating free radicals, also called reactive oxygen species. Free radicals are unstable molecules that damage cells, causing DNA damage that results in illness and ageing.

Sulforaphone (SFN) is a plant chemical that stimulates the body's natural antioxidant defences and detoxifying enzymes. SFN is a phytochemical produced when ingesting cruciferous vegetables containing glucoraphanin. Broccoli sprouts have the highest known amount of glucoraphanin, followed by other cruciferous vegetables – regular broccoli, cauliflower, cabbage and kale.

SFN can slow this ageing process as it activates the protective protein called NRF2, which is our most powerful antioxidant system. This stress adaptation system is built into all cells and constantly maintains the balance of internal oxidants to antioxidants. When robust, this system is capable of neutralising future exposures to many other stressors that increase free radicals and lead to damage. When there is an imbalance between free radicals and antioxidants in your body, that is when the body is in a state of oxidative stress.

Current research estimates that NRF2 is capable of upregulating 200+ genes that code for many roles in the body's defences against oxidative stress thus protecting our DNA and immunity.

NRF2 can also lower inflammation, boost the master antioxidant called glutathione, increase the number of mitochondria and support our cells' inbuilt detoxification system.

Pioneering researcher in this field, Dr Christine Houghton and some other scientists speculate this potent signal, within each of our trillions of cells, may have that healing power from within. The potential for far fewer supplements to achieve a powerful impact on the whole body comes from nature and sulphoraphane's power to activate NRF2.

Be careful with supplement quality though. Glucoraphanin can only be converted to sulforaphane with help from an enzyme called myrosinase. Myrosinase is activated when chewing, chopping, or crushing broccoli sprouts. However, myrosinase is deactivated when cooking broccoli sprouts, which washes out any potential for sulforaphane to activate NRF2 signalling.

Most people tell me they would prefer taking less supplements if they can still have great results. In my clinical work I've seen this impact numerous times through incorporating broccoli sprouts, as they activate so many core cellular pathways.

One remarkable story I witnessed was in a 41-year-old lady I worked with who had a long history of hormone imbalances and infertility who eventually fell pregnant at 41. Just six months prior, she started taking a clinician only supplement of broccoli sprouts and activated B vitamins that I had recommended to help her moods and hormones.

2. Magnesium

Magnesium facilitates over 300 different enzymatic reactions in the body and is especially important for our nervous system and energy production. Common symptoms of deficiency are fatigue, headaches, anxiety, depression, brain fog, heart palpitations, high blood pressure and insomnia. The vast majority of the population in the Western World is not consuming enough magnesium in their diets. The richest sources of the mineral are green leafy vegetables like silver beet (swiss chard in the US) and kale, followed by seeds such as pumpkin, hemp and chia. It can be challenging to obtain enough magnesium from food alone. Supplementation is valuable especially during stressful times in life, both to prevent deficiency and to maintain optimal levels.

The most common forms of magnesium support different processes in our body:

- Magnesium glycinate: Best for correcting overall magnesium deficiency. Also reduces anxiety and boosts relaxation and sleep quality.
- Magnesium citrate: Water-soluble form useful for many stress-related conditions, improving energy and alleviating constipation. Several recent studies comparing magnesium citrate with the magnesium oxide form (found in many retail supplements) found the citrate form provides significantly greater absorption.
- Magnesium threonate: Promotes calming signals for the nervous system as it can cross the blood-brain barrier. It is ideal for relieving brain fog, anxiety, improving focus and supporting sleep.

- Magnesium oxide is sometimes used as a short-term laxative as it is virtually insoluble (does not dissolve in water) and will rapidly empty the bowels. So it depends on the outcome you want to achieve, if you choose to take this form.
- Magnesium sulphate and magnesium chloride: Absorbed through the skin and not for oral ingestion. Epsom salts are common forms of magnesium sulphate. They are mainly used for soaking, soothing sore muscles and promoting relaxation.

3. Zinc

Zinc is an essential mineral and co-factor involved in over 300 different enzyme functions. Your nervous system, hormones, gut, wound healing and creation of new cells all require adequate zinc. It is quickly used up when experiencing a cold or flu, hormonal changes (i.e. puberty or menopause) or serious medical conditions. Most common zinc deficiencies can lead to poor sense of smell or taste, hyperactivity, aggression, hormone imbalances and frequent infections.

4. L-Theanine

L-Theanine is a natural amino acid and mild stimulant found in both green and black tea leaves. Green tea contains more beneficial plant compounds, up to 40 per cent water-soluble polyphenols, whereas black tea has only 3 to 10 per cent. The highest amount of L-theanine is found in ceremonial matcha green tea. Matcha coconut milk lattes have been part of my daily afternoon ritual for years, giving me clarity of mind and a calm, gentle energy lift.

By crossing the blood-brain barrier, L-Theanine can exert

neuroprotective effects to support two main calming neurotransmitters: GABA and serotonin. Increasing these neurotransmitters promotes relaxation and stress recovery. L-Theanine has been shown to improve memory and, with only a small amount of caffeine, it helps focus without jittery side effects from stronger stimulants. Research shows it can increase alpha-brain waves which encourage creativity and deep concentration. Optimal benefits for most people can come from drinking one cup (one serving) of matcha green tea per day with less than five servings recommended. Generally safe supplement dosages of L-Theanine range from 100 mg to 400 mg every six hours.

5. Omega 3 Fatty Acids

Fatty acids are the building blocks of *fat* in our bodies and in the foods we eat. Our brain is composed of 60 per cent fat. Fatty acids play a crucial role in influencing the function of membranes that serve as a protective 'skin' surrounding every brain cell. The kinds of fats and oils we eat are not at all equal.

If we often eat the wrong kind of fats, this imbalance can create excessive inflammation in our brain cells. Omega 3s are the anti-inflammatory fat our brains need for proper function and are considered to be essential fatty acids because our bodies cannot make them. So we need to consume them daily, from foods or in a high-purity supplement form.

These fatty acids are critical for memory, cognition, learning, mood and behaviour. Nutritionally, EPA (eicosapentaenoic acid) and DHA (docosahexaenoic acid) are the most important Omega 3 compounds. They reside in the cell membranes (outer layer) to exert their anti-inflammatory effects and keep our cells flexible. DHA and EPA have a unique function in the brain that contributes to our mental health. DHA is the form found in the brain. EPA boosts serotonin and regulates mood, while DHA makes up the cell membrane of neurotransmitters and enhances the expression of dopamine receptors.

Our mental health and cognitive function suffer when we have an excessive amount of trans fats or Omega-6s. The typical Western diet is overabundant in Omega 6s from processed foods, grains and oxidised nut- or seed- oils. Most diets contain a ratio of 15 to 1 Omega 6 to Omega 3, which is far from the recommended 4:1 ratio.

Omega 3s are also five times more sensitive to damage through heat, light and oxygen than Omega 6s. Our main source of EPA and DHA would be salmon (contains 2.208 grams DHA for 170gm/6oz fillet), sardines, herring or supplementation.

It is important to check your supplement brand independently tested the product to be free from plastics and heavy metals, as many fish oils are contaminated. Exposure to high temperatures can make fish oil supplements go rancid, so be sure to store yours in the fridge or a cool area away from heat and light. More recently a microalgae supplement has become available as a good vegetarian source of EPA and DHA.

6. Vitamin D

Vitamin D regulates the function of over 1000 different genes.

It is so much more than just a fat-soluble vitamin – it acts more like a hormone.

Nearly every cell inside our bodies has vitamin D receptors. These receptors bind to vitamin D and pull it into our cells. Once inside our cells, vitamin D binds to sites on our DNA that upregulate or downregulate our genes and regulate countless biological functions.

The function of our immune system, the strength of our bones, hormone and neurotransmitter production, and even cancer prevention depends on having enough vitamin D.

Achieving optimal vitamin D levels (100 mmol/ml) is a critical piece for chronic disease prevention. Skin exposure to sunshine is the most effective way to boost vitamin D levels. If you live somewhere that does not have a lot of sunshine or spend many days working indoors, I recommend a blood test and taking supplements if levels are low.

You might be surprised to know that, even in sunny climates the vast majority of people, even in Australia and the US have very low levels of this essential vitamin. It is wise to test Vitamin D levels at least once or twice a year.

7. Spirulina

Spirulina is a wild blue-green algae, considered by many researchers to be one of nature's most nutrient-dense superfoods.

It is most beneficial if you experience symptoms of excess heat or dryness in the body, such as constipation, heartburn or dehydration (even when drinking plenty of water).

It is ideal for taking during hot summer months as spirulina has "cooling" and "wet" properties. Daily consumption for women experiencing dryness, hot flushes and night sweats during perimenopausal years may be useful.

Spirulina is technically a food in powder form, so it is easy to add to smoothies or protein balls. This super algae is high in protein, beta carotene, nucleic acids and chlorophyll. The typical tablespoon (7gm) serving size delivers about 4gm of protein, so it can contribute towards daily protein intake, although would not be a main meal source.

It is also wonderfully alkalising for the body, although its taste can be unappealing for some. For this reason, it is readily available in blended powder formulas when mixed into smoothies, bliss balls or swallowed as capsules.

Suggested Dietary Guidelines

In our modern day, most people burn carbohydrates for fuel. Whether it is oats, a candy bar, bread, or pasta. These nutrients/ingredients are all broken down into simple sugars.

As humans, our ancestors did not have sugar or carbohydrates available every day and we are not designed to burn the high amount of sugar we use nowadays for fuel.

For many, our bodies have become used to burning these carbs without knowing what carb restriction does. Even though our bodies are well designed to burn fat for fuel. Our brains in particular thrive on ketones. These are produced when fasting, that is, going without food for at least 12 hours overnight. Our brains are wired to use fat as a fuel source, still with the mental clarity needed to focus in search of food when scarce. If possible switch your brain's fuel source from using sugars to more ketones (called ketosis). No matter what your age might be the benefits are numerous. My own clinical experience has consistently shown patient improvements in mood, focus, sleep, inflammation and detoxification come from regularly eating more vegetables alongside protein plus healthy fats with each meal.

I am not suggesting it is necessary to stay in ketosis consistently, forever restricting carbs for the rest of your life. However, having the dynamic ability to flexibly bounce back and forward with carbohydrate restriction is very healthy and supports long-term healing. This metabolic flexibility is how our bodies are pro-grammed to work, as in ancient times, sweet sugary foods were found only in seasonal fruit sources and are far less abundant than today. Having sugar or excessive amounts of carbohydrates every day is not what our brains and bodies are designed to run on. For this reason, a low-carb, high-fat (LCHF) eating approach is usually a good place to start if a ketogenic diet is too difficult.

12-week LCHF Nutritional Considerations

◆ Include 30gm of clean, unprocessed protein at every meal e.g. a combination of free-range eggs and chicken, grass-fed meat, wild salmon, sardines, non-GMO tofu or clean whey protein powder (organic is best).

◆ Aim to increase non-starchy and green leafy vegetables to about three to five cups per day for fibre and essential nutrients. Why this much and so specific? The latest research supports the wisdom our great-grandmothers would have said about "eating your vegetables". This principle is supported in a large review published in the 2021 journal *Circulation* from dozens of studies from around the world, which covered about 2 million people who were followed up to 30 years. Looking at all studies involved, the biggest health benefits came from eating leafy green vegetables (kale), fruits and vegetables rich in vitamin C and beta carotene (citrus, berries, carrots). No health benefit was recorded from eating starchy vegetables like peas, corn, or potatoes, or drinking fruit juice.

◆ Add in a daily tablespoon of cooked, stewed apple (ideally organic). Ayurveda has known benefits from eating stewed apples for thousands of years. Finally, recent studies have shown why; there is a type of gut bacteria that benefits from the apple-derived pectin.

◆ Initially avoid most grains, legumes and other high starchy carbohydrate foods to calm inflammation and eliminate common triggers for intestinal permeability.

◆ Include a generous portion of natural fats at each main meal. The best natural fats, depending on personal tolerance are: Ghee, butter, avocado, extra virgin olive oil, coconut milk, tahini, raw nuts and seeds. Tip: Pre-soak fresh nuts and seeds before eating for easier digestion. The best choices are pumpkin seeds, sunflower seeds or a sesame paste (tahini).

◆ Avoid hidden sugars and highly palatable processed foods and beverages, inclusive of dried fruit, acai bowls, and syrups (rice malt, maple, honey). Avoid all fruit juices, processed biscuits, cakes, candy, crackers and chips.

◆ Avoid folic acid-fortified foods (almost all commercial products made from wheat such as bread, pasta and baked goods), vegetable oils, fried foods and charred foods.

◆ Avoid high starch foods e.g. potatoes and grains as much as possible. Especially avoid gluten-containing grains (rye, wheat, barley, couscous etc.) and only occasionally eat organic oats if you tolerate them. Conventional oats in some countries for many years have been desiccated with harmful glyphosate weed killer to dry crops just before harvesting. Contaminated residue was detected in dozens of wheat and oat cereals in North American product testing. Organic oats have not been implicated in this practice.

◆ Avoid fermented foods and beverages e.g. yeast, cider, beer, sauerkraut, kimchi and kombucha. These histamine-rich foods can be fine if your brain is not already overstimulated. Histamine, like glutamate, is another excitatory neurotransmitter that is also released by stress. Some people do not clear histamine well due to variations in the DAO gene. Test it out by removing this cluster of foods for a while and see how you feel.

◆ Avoid all conventional casein-containing dairy, including lactose-free products, milk, yoghurt, cheese, and cream. Organic forms of butter, whey protein, kefir and natural yoghurt are well-tolerated by some. Thus there is no need to avoid them.

FOOD AND DRINKS LIST

FOODS TO ADD

Food Groups	Choose a variety of these daily
Low Starch Vegetables	Unlimited or at least 3 cups+: Bok choy, chives, cucumber, witlof, ginger, dino kale, cos lettuce, rocket, capsicum, silverbeet, radish, shallots, tomatoes, sunflower sprouts, alfalfa sprouts, eggplant, broccoli, zucchini, celery, cauliflower, fennel, wombok cabbage, green beans, snow peas. Prebiotic fibres best in small 1/4 cups serves from: Asparagus, brussel sprouts, artichokes, onions and garlic – if you are sensitive try the green ends of eshallots instead.
Root Vegetables	1/2-1 cup of either cooked pumpkin, carrots, beetroot, parsnips or sweet potato.
Fruits	1/2 cup per day of lemons, limes, blueberries, raspberries, kiwi, avocado (also a fat); or 1/2 cup of stewed apple or pear is tolerated by some too.
Low Starch Grains	1/2 cup per day: Buckwheat, quinoa, basmati rice or organic oats; ideally avoid if possible or limit to these serves if you do not want to remove grains just yet.
Meats and Fish	100-200gm: All additive free, grassfed or organic is best.
Nuts and Seeds	2 tbsp x 2 meals, approx. 40 nuts or 40gm daily of nut or seed butter from: Sunflower seeds, sesame seeds, poppy seeds, almonds, pistachios, macadamia nuts, pecans, pumpkin seeds, sunflower seeds, walnuts, hazelnuts and coconut flakes. Ideally soak whole nuts for easier digestion. Use seeds like chia or flaxseeds with caution if constipation prone. They are suitable for those with loose stools or normal digestion..
Herbs, Spices & Others	Parsley, coriander, mint, basil, rosemary, paprika, thyme, ginger, turmeric, cumin, oregano, sumac, Celtic salt, lemon juice, cinnamon, apple cider vinegar (ACV), spirulina, cacao, carob, cardamon, fennel seeds and vanilla (pure).
Fats & Oils	2 tbsp x 3 serves (about 60ml per day). Grass fed ghee, extra virgin olive oil, unrefined coconut oil, organic butter (if tolerated), olives, tahini and 1/2 avocado.
Beverages	Unlimited clean water, dandelion root, lemon, peppermint or ginger tea and black expresso coffee. Homemade drinks: Sparkling mineral water with drops of 'Sweet Leaf ' liquid stevia.1-2 cups of homemade hot or cold lattes using raw cacao, matcha or turmeric blend powder.

FOODS TO AVOID

Food Groups	
Vegetables	Corn, white potatoes and fermented foods such as sauerkraut and kimchi (high in histamine).
Fruits	All with the exception of fruit listed on the left.
Nuts and seeds	Peanuts are a high risk mycotoxin (mould-containing) as they are legumes, not true nuts.
Dairy and nondairy substitutes	Conventional cow, sheep and goat milk products (especially made as margarine, cream, yoghurt, ice cream, cheese and conventional whey); also most vegan protein powders.
Sweeteners	All inclusive of sugar, honey, maple syrup, rice malt, treacle, coconut sugar and dried fruit.
Beverages	Alcohol (especially beer, cider and wine), coconut water, kombucha, cordial, soft drinks, fruit and vegetable juices. If special events cannot avoid alcohol then best choices are vodka, gin and scotch with soda.
Legumes	All are best to avoid if possible or only have cooked mung beans.
Baking & Stocks	Yeast and breads made with the below flours.
Grains	Brown rice, arborio rice, wheat, spelt, barley, rye, kumut, couscous, millet and amaranth.

Sample Meal Plan

— 9 —

C.A.R.E. RECIPES

*"Eat your food like medicine otherwise you
have to eat medicine like food in the future"*
— Tapas Das

Healthy Ideas That Taste Delicious

Theses nutrient-packed recipes are designed to make foundational
healthy changes easier. All recipes are wheat-free, mostly paleo
and simple to modify for vegan or vegetarian options.

People sometimes tell me, they *"cannot afford healthy foods all
the time"* or that it is *"too expensive"*. What may be overlooked is
that processed, packaged, ready-to-eat food or fast food takeaways
and restaurant meals add up to being much more costly. Unless
you plan to eat lobster every week, home-cooked, healthy food
can save money. This style of eating is based on whole foods that
are more satisfying. Clinical experience with countless people I
have worked with feel full for longer and, with time, eat far fewer
snack foods than before.

Sample Meal Plan

Sample meal portions for one adult

At each meal of breakfast, lunch or dinner:

1-1.5 serve x protein/2 serves x fats/3 serves x veg/1x starchy carb

1 portion = ~120 grams protein (~4oz) animal or tofu

1 portion = 1/4 avocado or 1 tbsp of other fats (the size of your little finger)

1 portion = 1 cup non-starchy vegetables e.g. broccoli, dark kale or cabbage etc. (approx. 200gm x 3 with ideal total of ~600gm)

1 portion = 1/2 cup low sugar fruit or starchy carb (starchy veggies e.g. pumpkin, carrot or beetroot) or 1/2 cup of one cooked GF grain (e.g. basmati rice, buckwheat or quinoa)

....

Breakfasts

....

Super Green Protein Smoothie Bowl

1 scoop organic whey protein (vanilla is ideal)

1 cup greens (e.g. cos lettuce)

1/2 continental cucumber

1/2 cup unsweetened coconut milk, almond milk

or extra 1/2 cup of purified water

1/2 avocado

1/4 cup frozen blueberries

2 tbsp almond butter or similar

1 tbsp spirulina

1 tsp fresh lemon juice (optional)

Blend all together. Eat from a bowl for slower digestion and enjoyment. Enjoy immediately for the best flavour and nutrient value. Some separation is normal if kept in the fridge for a few hours.

Berry Cauli Protein Smoothie

1 cup cauliflower (precooked then frozen or frozen cauliflower rice)
1/2 cup unsweetened coconut milk or almond milk
1/4 avocado (makes it very creamy)
4 tbsp hemp or chia seeds
1 scoop organic whey protein powder (vanilla)
1/2 cup frozen or fresh berries of choice
Extra drops of liquid stevia, optional if more sweetness is desired.
Blend all together, except for seeds. Add seeds at the end of blending. Serve from a bowl to eat for slower digestion and enjoyment.

Fresh Lime Smoothie Bowl

1 scoop organic whey protein powder (vanilla works well)
1 handful of cos lettuce
1/2 frozen zucchini
1/2 lime (fresh juice)
1/4 cup coconut milk
2 tbsp cooked buckwheat (optional or omit if avoiding grains)
1 tbsp macadamias
1 tbsp fresh ginger
Blend all together and eat from a bowl for slower digestion and enjoyment.

Chocolate Smoothie Bowl

2 tbsp macadamias
2 tbsp raw cacao

1/2 cup unsweetened coconut milk or purified water

few drops of vanilla liquid stevia

Blend all together and eat from a bowl for slower digestion and enjoyment.

Almond Meal & Pumpkin Pudding

1 egg

1/4 – 1/2 cup of almond milk

1/4 cup of mashed pumpkin

2 tbsp of almond meal

1 tbsp unsweetened almond butter

1 tsp each of organic spices – cinnamon, ground ginger

few drops of vanilla liquid stevia (to taste)

Precook up a batch of pumpkin and mash to keep in the fridge. In a small bowl whisk egg and spices. Warm the pumpkin and almond meal in a saucepan. Add in the egg mix and stir quickly. Serve in a bowl with nut butter on top.

Zucchini Pancake

2 medium zucchini, grated or spiralised

3 free-range eggs

1/2 cup buckwheat flour (or 1/4 cup coconut flour)

1 tbsp olive oil or ghee for frying

Whisk eggs first. Blend all together in a bowl. Once the batter looks mixed pour into an oiled cast iron skillet or frying pan. Cook for 2 minutes on each side until light brown. Serve with the leafy greens of your choice.

Breakfast Bliss Balls

1 cup organic whey protein (vanilla or chocolate)
1/3 cup cacao powder
1/3 cup tahini or almond butter
1/2 cup shredded coconut
1/3 cup coconut flour or organic oats (if not gluten-free)
Few drops of liquid vanilla stevia to preferred taste

First mix coconut shreds in a food processor then add and blend all other ingredients until a dough has formed. Spoon out the dough and roll it into balls. Add a dash of water or more tahini/coconut butter if not sticking together well. Place on baking paper and store in the fridge for up to 1 week or 1 month in the freezer.

Vanilla Protein Cookies

2 cups organic buckwheat grouts, cooked (or rolled oats if tolerated)
1 cup (~4 scoops) organic vanilla whey protein powder
1/2 cup organic butter or ghee
1/2 cup almond meal
3/4 cup desiccated coconut
3/4 tsp bicarbonate of soda

Preheat your oven to 180°C/350°F (fan-forced). Line a small (approx. 20cm x 30cm) slice of tin with baking or parchment paper. In a medium-sized pot, heat the ghee (or butter) over low heat to melt. Mix in the bicarbonate of soda. Add the rest of the ingredients and mix well to combine. Add in liquid stevia drops (about 10) if you wish to increase sweetness. Place into the oven for 20 to 30 minutes or until golden brown on top. The longer you cook it, the crisper the cookies become. Allow to cool and store sealed in the refrigerator.

Lunch or Dinners

Ginger Coconut Salmon (1 serve)

150gm wild-caught salmon fillet (fresh or frozen)

Marinade for each salmon fillet (min 1-hour or overnight) in:

1/3 cup coconut milk

1 tbsp coconut aminos or tamari

1/2tsp ginger

1/4 tsp turmeric, pinch of pepper and salt

Olive oil, butter or ghee if pan frying

Grill or pan fry in butter or oil for 10 to 15 minutes or oven bake at 180°C. Serve with 1 cup of any cooked green veggies and 1/2 cup of cooked carrots. Carrot and ginger are delicious in the same meal.

Clean & Easy Salmon Patties (serves 2)

1 x 400gm Alaskan tinned salmon (with mashed bones for calcium)

1 cup cooked cauliflower

1/2 cup buckwheat flour (or 1/4 cup coconut flour)

2 tbsp lemon juice and a pinch of Himalayan salt

Mix and mash well all ingredients in a saucepan or mixing bowl. Make into patty shapes. Fry in a little ghee or olive oil until brown on both sides. Just add cooked greens of your choice on the side. Can be frozen for up to one month after completely cooling.

Beef Veggie Hash (4 serves)

1 tbsp olive oil or ghee

1 small onion (chopped)

2 cloves garlic (minced)

1/2 tsp cinnamon

1 tsp ground ginger

1 tsp turmeric

1/2 tsp sea salt

500gm beef mince (grass-fed or organic preferably)

2 medium carrots or pumpkin (bite-sized precooked is easiest)

1 bunch of kale leaves (chopped)

1 tbsp lemon juice (fresh)

In a cast iron skillet, heat olive oil over medium heat. Add onions and cook until softened and becoming translucent. About 5 minutes. Stir in garlic, cinnamon, ginger, turmeric and salt. Cook until fragrant, about 1 minute. Immediately add ground beef. Break up beef as it cooks with a wooden spoon and stir as needed. When beef is quite cooked through, add orange root veggies and cook, continuing to stir frequently until is softened. About 5-7 minutes. Stir in kale and allow to cook until wilted and softened. About 3 minutes. Check carrot/pumpkin for the softness desired. Stir in lemon juice. Taste and add more salt if desired.

Sauces and Sides

Creamed Kale

5 cups dark green kale or silver beet

1/2 cup full-fat coconut milk (AYAM brand or other BPA-free)

3 tbsp ghee or extra virgin olive oil

3 tbsp shallots

2 tsp tamari or coconut aminos

1/2 tsp minced fresh ginger

1/4 tsp Himalayan salt

Heat oil in a cast iron skillet and add all ingredients except for coconut milk and aminos. Cook for 2–3 mins or until kale wilts. Stir coconut milk in; cover and cook for 2–4 mins until kale is tender. Serve warm.

Creamy Carrot Soup

5 cups bone broth (or 5 tsp broth concentrate equivalent)

2 cups cooked red onion

700gm diced carrots

250ml coconut milk

2 chopped celery stalks

1 tsp turmeric powder

2 tsp curry powder

1/2 tsp minced fresh ginger

1/2 tsp ground cumin

1/2 tsp pink salt

Heat oil in a cast iron skillet and add pan-fry onions, carrot, celery and garlic. Saute for 7 minutes until the onions become soft. Add turmeric, curry powder, cumin and salt. Mix for 1 minute more. Add broth and coconut milk into a saucepan then stir. Close the pot and lock the lid. Set to high pressure and cook for 5 mins. Using a stick blender, blend the soup to the desired consistency. Serve with an extra dollop of coconut milk or cream.

"Herbal Detox" Salsa

3 handfuls of fresh organic herbs; one each

of fresh parsley, basil and coriander (or mint)

1 cup of raw pre-soaked pumpkin seeds

1 lemon (juice only) or 1/2 cup premix to your taste

2 tbsp extra-virgin olive oil

2 tbsp tahini

1 tbsp apple cider vinegar

1 tsp fresh garlic, minced and organic is best (optional)

1/2 tsp turmeric organic powder

1/2 tsp Himalayan sea salt or to taste

1/2 cup nutritional yeast flakes

1/4 tsp cumin powder

1/8 tsp cayenne pepper (optional)

Blend pumpkin seeds then add one handful of each organic herbs. Combine all in a food processor or blender with the lemon juice, oil, tahini, all spices, salt and cayenne pepper. Process all ingredients, stopping to scrape down the sides of the bowl occasionally, until the mixture is smooth and begins to hold together. Add water or more lemon juice for a thinner consistency. Store in glass jars in the fridge for up to five days or freeze for up to one month. Enjoy with veggie sticks such as cucumber or add as a base sauce to any vegetable or salad bowl mix for extra flavour punch.

Leftover Mix-Ups – Light Lunches or Dinners

Handy Home Wrap

1 NuCo coconut wrap (GF)

1 cup cooked chicken breast or tinned salmon

1 cup cooked kale, silver beet or lettuce

2 tbsp homemade 'herbal detox' salsa

Spread protein and vegetables of choice onto centre of the coconut wrap. Roll up and enjoy.

Meaty Roast Veg Bowl

4 cups of vegetables of your choice, each week:
Beetroot, cauliflower, zucchini, eggplant, pumpkin, carrots, sweet
potato or fennel etc.
1 handful fresh herbs
1 handful pumpkin seeds or sunflower seeds
1 lemon or lime
1 tbspn olive oil

Meal prep a day or two before eating. Batch roast all vegetables of choice. Store ready in fridge. On day of eating or one day before cook your protein of choice. In a large bowl or container, add 1-2 cups of precooked vegetables. Add to this your cooked protein and a handful of chopped fresh herbs. Drizzle all with lemon or lime juice and olive oil. Add a handful of sunflower or seeds for crunch.

Seaside Macro Bowl

1 cup of cooked greens such as sautéed zucchini, cabbage or green beans
1/2 cup cos lettuce or rocket (arugula)
1/2 cup mashed pumpkin or carrots
1 cup salmon, mackerel or sardines
1 tbsp macadamia nut or almond butter
1 lemon

In one large bowl, combine all ingredients, except for nut butter and lemon. Drizzle nut butter and squeeze of lemon to finish.

Nourishing Treats (LCHF rewards)

Hot Cacao or Turmeric Collagen Drink

1 cup almond or coconut milk, heated

2 tsp collagen or protein powder

1 tbsp raw cacao (or 1 tsp turmeric spice blend)

Drops of liquid stevia as desired (or 1 tsp monk fruit)

Blend all together and pour into a mug to enjoy.

Blueberry Cream Gummies

400 ml canned full fat coconut milk

1 cup blueberries (frozen then defrosted)

1 cup boiling water

10 vanilla stevia drops- or 1 tsp vanilla essence

4 tbsp grass-fed gelatin

In a small saucepan, heat the coconut milk over low heat (avoid boiling it). Add 2 tablespoons of the gelatin to 2 tablespoons of cold water and allow it to bloom. Mix together with a spoon. Add gelatin to the coconut milk and stir until all lumps are gone. In a high-speed blender, blend the blueberries until a pulp forms. Add the boiling water and vanilla stevia to the blender, blend again then add the remaining 2 tablespoons of gelatin and process until the gelatin has dissolved. Pour the coconut milk layer into a deep-lined dish or ceramic container. Then gently pour over the slayer (swirling as you pour creates the pattern on the top). Pop into the fridge for about 30 minutes to set. Slice and enjoy.

Zesty Lemon Protein Balls

1 cup macadamia nuts (pre-soaked overnight)

1 cup (approx. 4 scoops) vanilla organic whey protein

1/4 cup coconut (organic desiccated or shredded)

1 lemon (juice and zest)

2 tbsp ghee or tahini

2 tsp spirulina

Water (if needed to combine dry and wet ingredients)

Blend all together and pour the mixture into a lined dish. Freeze for one hour, then cut into bite sizes. Separate once hardened from the freezer.

Crunchy Almond Stewed Apples

2 organic apples (Granny Smith or other firm variety)

1 scoop vanilla organic whey protein (or similar)

1/3 cup water

1/4 cup sunflower seeds or similar for crunch

1 tsp cinnamon

1/4 cup almond butter

Core the apples and slice into rough cubes. Add apples and water to small saucepan. Bring to boil, then reduce to medium heat for about 5 minutes with lid on. Watch the water doesn't all disappear. Add cinnamon towards the end. Allow apple mix to cool completely. Pour into a storage dish and add protein powder for a thicker texture. Drizzle almond butter and sunflower seeds over the top and place in fridge for later or enjoy right away. Serves 1 or 2 people.

Troubleshooting – Why Still Having Cravings?

◆ You want a healthy dopamine hit – try exercise, a cold water plunge or shower, dancing, meditation, sex and intimacy.

If you have some addictive risk genes mentioned in Chapter 6 these simple tips may help: Choose snacks that address different sensory aspects of the mouth, such as texture (chewy, crunchy or crispy) and other flavours from herbs and spices. The more sensory profiles a snack has the more satisfied and less likely you will keep snacking or grazing. To avoid getting hungry between meals it is best to eat three main meals a day that include protein, healthy fat and fibre from an unlimited amount of low-starchy veggies (roasted vegetables are my favourites). See Chapter 9 for easy, creative recipe ideas.

◆ If you have not slept well or enough this pattern changes your appetite-regulating hormones, ghrelin and leptin. Less than 6.5 hours a night will also increase blood sugar levels. Eating clean on this kind of day is best and takes quite some effort. I see success in many when they focus on unlimited amounts of roasted vegetables, soups or vegetable smoothies alongside their favourite protein for those days they lack sleep. Then go to bed as early as you can the next night.

- You have skipped meals – this decreases blood sugar levels that can leave you screaming for a sugar hit if lingering too long. Please keep to a regular meal routine for a few weeks to establish that feeling of safety in your body.

- You have got PMS – do not fight it. Make nourishing, filling meals and if due that day have some dark chocolate. It will be a pleasurable small reward.

- You have food sensitivities – this alters brain chemistry and depresses serotonin levels, as serotonin is called in to counter inflammation that consuming food-sensitive foods like gluten and casein (in dairy). Eliminating gluten and dairy foods allows your brain's serotonin levels to rise naturally, providing you access to all the serotonin your brain synthesizes.

- Your last meal was too salty – a balanced flavour contains fat, acid, salt and sweet – F.A.S.S. for short. If one element is overly dominant, you will crave flavour that was submissive in the meal, most commonly the sweetener. The antidote for this is not sugar. Water or sour flavours like lemon will dilute the saltiness. Have a glass of sparkling water instead of dessert. A better way of nurturing yourself after dinner is a warm cup of tea or cooled herbal tea.

Don't Know What's Working?

Be mindful of what you are eating and how you feel hours afterwards.

Temporarily recording data can be a powerful way to identify foods that do not agree with you and find substitute foods that do.

Some people like to take notes on their phones or use pen and paper or an app to track their food and mood. List what you ate or drank, and a few words that describe how you feel overall. Rate your mood from 0 to 10, where zero is pretty awful and 10 is feeling great. Write as much or as little as you can.

A fuller food diary tracker maps out more details to include moods, bowel movements, sleep, stress and energy levels with food and drinks eaten is best. See the resources section to download an editable template. There are also many free online food and symptom tracking apps for smartphones, such as *Cara Care* or *Foody – Food and Symptom* Tracker.

If tracking makes you feel more stressed, don't worry. Focus on eating less processed foods, more vegetables and home-cooked meals. Perhaps tracking may be useful later on.

C.A.R.E. in Practice

Reaching this part of the book means you have likely identified some of the genetic traits and causative factors for feeling overwhelmed from Part 1.

Interpreting the meaning behind your mind-body signals that correspond with genes that fuel the needs of your gut, brain and behavioural patterns was explored in Part 2. In Part 3, I offered some lifestyle strategies and the C.A.R.E. framework to implement activities and an eating method to help feel stronger and speed up healing.

There are many simple actions you can try when ready to make a start, no matter where you are at right now. If you are ready to experiment then perhaps add in a new recipe or healthier food from the list or start with an activity that looks appealing.

Suggested Sequential Steps:

1. Identify your current signals of discomfort and use insight from the <u>factors in the overwhelm map</u> from Chapter 1 to ask, "*What I can control?*"

2. Interpret deeper signals you are currently having in any or all of the <u>gut, brain and behaviour areas</u> alongside traits of these genes. When combining this understanding of these layers you can start to see where to focus attention first. Ask yourself, "What's realistic for now?" and "How can I correct this pattern in the most urgent areas?"

3. Implement some of the lifestyle activities, supplements and/or food changes as a 12 week experiment to simultaneously support your mind–body signals alongside your priority gene pathways.

You have the power and potential within you once you know how to take control of your health. Who you uniquely are, based on patterns stored in your DNA alongside feedback from your mind and body, is a valuable insight for functioning your best and being free from the one-size-fits-all approach to healing. You will gain confidence to trust your intuition and connect with the right social environment.

Learning how to re-regulate your nervous system and support all gene pathways will help you quickly return to feeling balanced, no matter what life throws at you. It will take time, and some experimentation to learn what works best for you and how your body responds.

When you respond with awareness rather than react to your situation, you can take the driver's seat to adopt better behaviours and reach your health potential. You may even notice the simple pleasures in life once again. This awareness gives you more control over daily actions and the ability to think differently. It is a process that moves you from feeling powerless to empowered.

Every input we have coming through our senses impacts not only how we look but how we feel in the process. Sometimes, problems seem far too complicated to be helped by simple things like good food, regular physical movement and sleep. Tracking your daily inputs can help upgrade your new habits with confidence and see what works and what does not. Ask better questions helps. Something like, *"What's the next obstacle(s) I need to overcome?"*

FINAL WORDS

Moving You from Powerless to Empowered

Thank you for joining me on this journey, which hopefully gives you clarity and clear strategies that will help you move from feeling powerless to more powerful and empowered towards freedom. I wish you good health, peace and happiness. Take heart in knowing that no matter what falls happen along the way, you can begin again, anytime, in supporting the foundations of your mind and body.

APPENDIX

Genetic Testing

Many DNA genetic testing companies offer direct-to-consumer genetic tests that take just 60 sec to do as a simple cheek swab at home. It is not a pathology test (like blood, stool or urine) that continuously changes throughout our lives. As your genes never change it is a one-time-only test. Your DNA test will not diagnose any particular health condition. Gene marker variants only indicate the probability of specific health risks. The quality of lab technology, privacy standards and the genes they report vary widely.

The best value will come from a testing lab that highlights genes from core biochemical pathways with clinical usefulness. Test prices vary from around $200–$500. Working with an accredited nutrigenomics practitioner who can analyse and interpret your genetic test results can provide optimal guidance for better health and balance. Overall, there is so much to gain from knowing both your risky genes and strong ones. You control the influence of how your genes work. See the resources list for test and interpretation recommendations.

Terms

Gene – a basic molecular and functional unit that is passed down from ancestors, one generation to the next.

Genome – an individual's complete set of genetic information.

DNA – deoxyribonucleic acid, contains the code or pattern information to instruct cells and all of the molecules that make us unique.

Polymorphism – variations of a gene code, sometimes called SNPs that may determine differences between individual height, eye colour or behavioural traits.

Gene variation (not a mutation) – a permanent change in the DNA sequence that may be inherited or occur spontaneously during cell division.

RESOURCES

If you are interested to find out more about this mind and body approach to health, the related self-help tools and organisations in the following list can offer support. No financial relationship is linked with any of these.

Websites

- ACE – adverse childhood events questionnaire – Accessed 2024. https://www.acesaware.org/wp-content/uploads/2020/02/ACE-Questionnaire-for-Adults-Identified-English.pdf
- CGM – Continuous glucose monitor. Accessed 2024. https://www.levelshealth.com/blog/what-is-a-continuous-glucose-monitor
- Diet-based approach clinician directory for addressing metabolic dysfunction for mental health. Accessed 2024. https://www.diagnosisdiet.com/directory
- Food and symptom diary – Accessed 2024. https://fill.io/Orthoplex-DIET-and-SYMPTOM-DIARY
- Falun Dafa Information Center. Ancient Roots, Almost Lost. 2015a. https://faluninfo.net/falun-gong-story-ancient-roots
- HSP test – Accessed 2024. https://hsperson.com/test/highly-sensitive-test
- Institute for Nutrigenomic Medicine: Specialists trained in nutritional genomics. https://nutrigenomicmedicine.com
- Genetics test: 3x4 Genetics for lifestyle genomics test and expert trained nutrigenomic practitioners. https://3x4genetics.com

- Nutrition Network, global directory of accredited practitioners trained in Therapeutic Carbohydrate Restriction. Accessed 2024. https://nutrition-network.org/find-a-practitioner
- Meditation links – Falun Data meditation and qigong exercises worldwide. https://faluninfo.net/what-is-falun-gong-falun-dafa
- Polyvagal Regulation – Accessed 2024. https://www.rhythmofregulation.com
- S.U.G.A.R. Addiction protocol – Accessed 2024. https://www.bittensaddiction.com/en/patients/certified-licensed-sugar-professionals
- Sugar Addiction support online group – Accessed 2024. https://www.sugarxglobal.com
- YALE Food addiction scale. https://sites.lsa.umich.edu/fastlab/yale-food-addiction-scale or https://www.psychologyunlocked.com/yale-food-addiction-scale (with 35 questions to help us define what it means to struggle with food).

Books

Van der Kolk, Bessel A., *The Body Keeps the Score: Brain, Mind, and Body in the Healing of Trauma*

Clear, James, *Atomic Habits*

Houghton, Dr Christine, *Switched On: Embracing the Science of Nutrigenomic Medicine*

Joffe, Dr Yael, *The Power Of Genetics: DNA, daily decisions, and the journey to taking control of your health*

Kumai, Candice, *Kintsugi Wellness*

Li Hongzhi. *Zhuan Falun.* Taipei, Taiwan; Yih Chyun Book Co. Ltd; 2014

Lo, Imi, *Emotional Sensitivity and Intensity: How to manage emotions as a highly sensitive person*

Nestor, James, *Breath*

Orloff, Dr Judith, *The Empath's Survival Guide*

Porges, Dr Stephen, *The Polyvagal Theory*

Trey, Margaret, *The Mindful Practice of Falun Gong: Meditation for Health, Wellness and Beyond.* [2nd edition]. Otisville, NY: Sibubooks LLC; 2020

Notes

Chapter 1

Mate, Gabor. When the Body Says No: The cost of hidden stress (2019) ISBN: 9781925849646

Sterling P, Eyer J. Allostasis: a new paradigm to explain arousal pathology. In: Fisher S, Reason HS, editors.*Handbook of Life Stress Cognition and Health.*\New York: Wiley; 1981.

Dunn, B. D., Galton, H. C., Morgan, R., Evans, D., Oliver, C., Meyer, M., Dalgleish, T. (2010). Listening to your heart: How interoception shapes emotion experience and intuitive decision making. *Psychological Science,**21,* 1835.\https://doi.org/10.1177/0956797610389191

Levine, Peter. Waking the Tiger; Healing Trauma (2011), ISBN: 9781556432330
Bessel A. Van Der Kolk,\The Body Keeps the Score: Brain, Mind, and Body in the Healing of Trauma\(2015), ISBN: 9780141978611

Kumai, Candice. Kintsugi Wellness: The Japanese Art of Nourishing Mind, Body, and Spirit (2018); ISBN: 0062669850

DNA definition. Accessed 2024: https://www.science.org.au/curious/people-medicine/human-genome-project

Colvis CM, Pollock JD, Goodman RH, Impey S, Dunn J, Mandel G, Champagne FA, Mayford M, Korzus E, Kumar A, Renthal W, Theobald DE, Nestler EJ. Epigenetic mechanisms and gene networks in the nervous system. J Neurosci. 2005 Nov 9;25(45):10379-89. doi: 10.1523/JNEU-ROSCI.4119-05.2005. PMID: 16280577; PMCID: PMC6725821.

Clear, James. Atomic Habits; An Easy and Proven Way to Build Good Habits and Break Bad Ones (2018) ISBN: 9781847941831
emotions & organs. Accessed 2024: https://plato.stanford.edu/entries/emotions-chinese/

Chapter 2

Soares CN, Joffe H, Steiner M. Menopause and mood. Clin Obstet Gynecol. 2004 Sep;47(3):576-91. doi: 10.1097/01.grf.0000129918.00756.d5. PMID: 15326420.

https://nypost.com/2019/02/22/nearly-half-of-women-have-been-affected-by-a-hormonal-imbalance/ — Accessed 2024

Monteleone, P., Mascagni, G., Giannini, A.*et al.*\Symptoms of menopause — global prevalence, physiology and implications.*Nat Rev Endocrinol*\14, 199–215 (2018). https://doi.org/10.1038/nrendo.2017.180

Brady CW. Liver disease in menopause. World J Gastroenterol. 2015 Jul 7;21(25):7613-20. doi: 10.3748/wjg.v21.i25.7613. PMID: 26167064; PMCID: PMC4491951.

Former Thong Chai Medical Institution - Home to the first free TCM medical clinic in SG to assist low-income people.
https://www.roots.gov.sg/en/stories-landing/stories/history-of-healthcare-sg — Accessed 2024:

Lustig, Robert, MD. Metabolical (2023), ISBN: 9781529350074

Chapter 3
Aaron, Elaine. PhD. THE HIGHLY SENSITIVE PERSON: How to Thrive When the World Over-whelms You; (2017) ISBN: 0-553-06218-2

Kibe, C., Suzuki, M., Hirano, M., etal...Boniwell, I. (2020). Sensory processing sensitivity and culturally modified resilience education: Differential susceptibility in Japanese adoles-cents.*PloS one*, 15(9), e0239002.

Shuhei Iimura;\Sensory-processing sensitivity and COVID-19 stress in a young population: The mediating role of resilience Pers Individ Dif 2022 Jan;184:111183. doi: 10.1016/j.paid.2021.111183. Epub 2021 Aug 9.

Orloff, Judith; The Empath's Survival Guide: Life Strategies for Sensitive People (2019) ISBN: 9781683642114

IBS Study on HSPs - Int. J. Environ. Res. Public Health 2022, 19(16), 9893;\https://doi.org/10.3390/ijerph19169893

Lo, Imi;\Emotional Sensitivity and Intensity: How to manage emotions as a highly sensitive person\(2018) ISBN: 9781473656031

Bianca P Acevedo,1\Elaine N Aron. The highly sensitive brain: an fMRI study of sensory pro-cessing sensitivity and response to others' emotions;\Brain Behav.\2014 Jul; 4(4): 580–594. https://www.ncbi.nlm.nih.gov/pmc/articles/PMC4086365/

Chapter 4
Wardlaw, G. and Insel, P.*Perspectives in Nutrition*, (2001) ISBN: 0072489405
Disorders. Accessed 2024: https://theromefoundation.org/what-is-a-disorder-of-gut-brain-interaction-dgbi/
IBS Prevalence. Accessed 2024: https://aboutibs.org/

Breit S, Kupferberg A, Rogler G, Hasler G. Vagus Nerve as Modulator of the Brain-Gut Axis in

Psychiatric and Inflammatory Disorders. Front Psychiatry. 2018 Mar 13;9:44. doi: 10.3389/ fpsyt.2018.00044. PMID: 29593576; PMCID: PMC5859128.

What is a leaky gut? Fasano A. All disease begins in the (leaky) gut: role of zonulin-mediated gut permeability in the pathogenesis of some chronic inflammatory diseases. F1000Res. 2020 Jan 31;9:F1000 Faculty Rev-69. doi: 10.12688/f1000research.20510.1. PMID: 32051759; PMCID: PMC6996528.

Porges, Stephen PhD. The Polyvagal Theory: Neurophysiological Foundations of Emotions, Attachment, Communication, and Self-regulation (2011); ISBN: 0393707008
Nestor, James, Breath: The new science of a lost art, (2020); ISBN: 0735213615

Perlmutter, David & Austin. MDs. Brain Wash (2020) ISBN: 0316453323

MTHFR

Leclerc D, Sibani S, Rozen R. Molecular Biology of Methylenetetrahydrofolate Reductase (MTHFR) and Overview of Mutations/Polymorphisms. In: Madame Curie Bioscience Database [Internet]. Austin (TX): Landes Bioscience; 2000-2013. Available from: https://www.ncbi.nlm. nih.gov/books/NBK6561/

What is Folate? Accessed 2024: https://ods.od.nih.gov/factsheets/Folate-HealthProfessional/

Levin BL, Varga E. MTHFR: Addressing Genetic Counseling Dilemmas Using Evidence-Based Literature. J Genet Couns. 2016 Oct;25(5):901-11. doi: 10.1007/s10897-016-9956-7. Epub 2016 Apr 30. PMID: 27130656.

FTO

Frayling TM, Timpson NJ et.al. A common variant in the FTO gene is associated with body mass index and predisposes to childhood and adult obesity. Science. 2007 May 11;316(5826):889-94. doi: 10.1126/science.1141634. Epub 2007 Apr 12. PMID: 17434869; PMCID: PMC2646098.

Szalanczy, A. et al. Genetic variation in satiety signaling and hypothalamic inflammation: merging fields for the study of obesity, The Journal of Nutritional Biochemistry, Volume 101,2022,108928, ISSN 09552863, https://doi.org/10.1016/j.jnutbio.2021.108928.

Speliotes EK, et al. Association analyses of 249,796 individuals reveal 18 new loci associated with body mass index.\Nat Genet.\2010;42(11):937–948. doi: 10.1038/ng.686.

CLOCK

Functions of COMT gene. Accessed 2024: https://www.ncbi.nlm.nih.gov/gene/9575

Summa KC, Turek FW. Chronobiology and obesity: Interactions between circadian rhythms and energy regulation. Adv Nutr. 2014 May 14;5(3):312S-9S. doi: 10.3945/an.113.005132. PMID: 24829483; PMCID: PMC4013188.

Antypa N, Mandelli L, Nearchou FA, Vaiopoulos C, Stefanis CN, Serretti A, Stefanis NC. The 311T/C polymorphism interacts with stressful life events to influence patterns of sleep in females. Chronobiol Int. 2012 Aug;29(7):891-7. doi: 10.3109/07420528.2012.699380. PMID: 22823872

Chapter 5
Stephen W. Porges,*The Polyvagal Theory: Neurophysiological Foundations of Emotions, Attachment, Communication, Self-regulation*, Norton Series on Interpersonal Neurobiology, New York, NY: W. W. Norton, April 2011;\"Science of Safety" – Polyvagal theory)

Dana, Deborah. Polyvagal Flip Chart: Understanding the Science of Safety (2020); ISBN: 0393714721
HSPs & anxiety. Soodan, S., & Arya, A. (2015). Understanding the pathophysiology and management of anxiety disorders. International Journal of Pharmacy & Pharmaceutical Research, 4(3), 251-278.

Benham, G.(2006) The Highly Sensitive Person: Stress and physical symptom reports. Personality and Individual Differences.Vol40. Issue 7. ISSN 0191-8869. https://doi.org/10.1016/j.paid.2005.11.021.

Brain Energy-Fuel supply.\Accessed 2024: https://pubmed.ncbi.nlm.nih.gov/12149485/

Fitzgerald, K. MD. Younger You: Reduce Your Bio Age and Live Longer, Better (2022), ISBN-10: 0274801795 DNA & cytokines. p217.

GI distress & HSPs. Iimura, S.; Takasugi, S. Sensory Processing Sensitivity and Gastrointestinal Symptoms in Japanese Adults.\Int. J. Environ. Res. Public Health\2022,\19, 9893. https://doi.org/10.3390/ijerph19169893

What is DGBI?\Accessed 2024: https://theromefoundation.org/what-is-a-disorder-of-gut-brain-interaction-dgbi/
Orloff, Judith; The Empath's Survival Guide: Life Strategies for Sensitive People (2019) ISBN: 9781683642114

ABDRA2B
Xie W, Cappiello M, Meng M, Rosenthal R, Zhang W. ADRA2B deletion variant and enhanced cognitive processing of emotional information: A meta-analytical review. Neurosci Biobehav Rev. 2018 Sep;92:402-416. doi: 10.1016/j.neubiorev.2018.05.010. Epub 2018 May 8. PMID: 29751052.

Todd RM, Müller DJ, Lee DH, Robertson A, Eaton T, Freeman N, Palombo DJ, Levine B, Anderson AK. Genes for emotion-enhanced remembering are linked to enhanced perceiving. Psychol Sci. 2013 Nov 1;24(11):2244-53. doi: 10.1177/0956797613492423. Epub 2013 Sep 20. PMID: 24058067.

COMT

Functions of COMT gene. Accessed 2024: https://medlineplus.gov/genetics/gene/comt/

Tiihonen J, Hallikainen T, Lachman H, Saito T, Volavka J, Kauhanen J, Salonen JT, Ryynänen OP, Koulu M, Karvonen MK, Pohjalainen T, Syvälahti E, Hietala J. Association between the functional variant of the catechol-O-methyltransferase (COMT) gene and type 1 alcoholism. Mol Psychiatry. 1999 May;4(3):286-9. doi: 10.1038/sj.mp.4000509. PMID: 10395222.

Enoch, M. A., Xu, K., Ferro, E., Harris, C. R., & Goldman, D. (2003). Genetic origins of anxiety in women: a role for a functional catechol-O-methyltransferase polymorphism.*Psych Genet,*13(1), 33-41.

Olsson, C. A., Anney, R. J., Lotfi-Miri, M., Byrnes, G. B., Williamson, R., & Patton, G. C. (2005). Association between the COMT Val158Met polymorphism and propensity to anxiety in an Australian population-based longitudinal study of adolescent health.*Psych Genet,*15(2), 109-115.

Witte, A. V., & Flöel, A. (2012). Effects of COMT polymorphisms on brain function and behavior in health and disease.*Brain Research Bulletin,*88(5), 418-428.

Antypa, N., Drago, A., & Serretti, A. (2013). The role of COMT gene variants in depression: Bridging neuropsychological, behavioral and clinical phenotypes.*Neuro Biobehav Rev,*37(8), 1597-1610.

BNDF

Leal G, Bramham CR, Duarte CB. BDNF and Hippocampal Synaptic Plasticity. Vitam Horm. 2017;104:153-195. doi: 10.1016/bs.vh.2016.10.004. Epub 2016 Nov 29. PMID: 28215294.

Miranda, M., Morici, J. F., Zanoni, M. B., & Bekinschtein, P. (2019). Brain-derived neurotrophic factor: a key molecule for memory in the healthy and the pathological brain.*Frontiers in Cellular Neuroscience*, 363.

Numakawa T, Odaka H, Adachi N. Actions of Brain-Derived Neurotrophic Factor and Glucocorticoid Stress in Neurogenesis. Int J Mol Sci. 2017 Nov 2;18(11):2312. doi: 10.3390/ijms18112312. PMID: 29099059; PMCID: PMC5713281.

Rybakowski JK, Borkowska A, Czerski PM, Skibińska M, Hauser J. Polymorphism of the brain-derived neurotrophic factor gene and performance on a cognitive prefrontal test in bipolar patients. Bipolar Disord. 2003 Dec;5(6):468-72. doi: 10.1046/j.1399-5618.2003.00071.x. PMID: 14636373.

Bus, B., Molendijk, M., Tendolkar, I.\et al.\Chronic depression is associated with a pronounced decrease in serum brain-derived neurotrophic factor over time.\Mol Psychiatry\20, 602–608 (2015). https://doi.org/10.1038/mp.2014.83

Cattaneo, A., Cattane, N., Begni, V.\et al.\The human BDNF gene: peripheral gene expression and protein levels as biomarkers for psychiatric disorders.\Transl Psychiatry\6, e958 (2016). https://doi.org/10.1038/tp.2016.214

Gagrani M, Faiq MA, Sidhu T, Dada R, Yadav RK, Sihota R, Kochhar KP, Verma R, Dada T. Meditation enhances brain oxygenation, upregulates BDNF and improves quality of life in patients with primary open angle glaucoma: A randomized controlled trial. Restor Neurol Neurosci. 2018;36(6):741-753. doi: 10.3233/RNN-180857. PMID: 30400122.

You T, Ogawa EF. Effects of meditation and mind-body exercise on brain-derived neurotrophic factor: A literature review of human experimental studies. Sports Med Health Sci. 2020 Mar 20;2(1):7-9. doi: 10.1016/j.smhs.2020.03.001. PMID: 35783336; PMCID: PMC9219319.

Chapter 6
Richard J.\Rosenthal\&\Suzanne B.\Faris\(2019)\The etymology and early history of 'addiction',\Addiction Research & Theory,\27:5,\437-449,\DOI:\10.1080/16066359.2018.1543412

Ifland JR, Preuss HG, Marcus MT, Rourke KM, Taylor WC, Burau K, Jacobs WS, Kadish W, Manso G. Refined food addiction: a classic substance use disorder. Med Hypotheses. 2009 May;72(5):518-26. doi: 10.1016/j.mehy.2008.11.035. Epub 2009 Feb 14. PMID: 19223127.

Lembke, Anna. MD. Dopamine Nation: Finding Balance in the Age of Indulgence (2023); ISBN: 1524746746

Epstein LH, Temple JL, Neaderhiser BJ, Salis RJ, Erbe RW, Leddy JJ. Food reinforcement, the dopamine D2 receptor genotype, and energy intake in obese and nonobese humans. Behav Neurosci. 2007 Oct;121(5):877-86. doi: 10.1037/0735-7044.121.5.877. Erratum in: Behav Neurosci. 2008 Feb;122(1):250. PMID: 17907820; PMCID: PMC2213752.

Doehring A, Kirchhof A, Lötsch J. Genetic diagnostics of functional variants of the human dopamine D2 receptor gene. Psychiatr Genet. 2009 Oct;19(5):259-68. doi: 10.1097/ YPG.0b013e32832d0941. PMID: 19512960.

Fenech M, El-Sohemy A, Cahill L, Ferguson LR, French TA, Tai ES, Milner J, Koh WP, Xie L, Zucker M, Buckley M, Cosgrove L, Lockett T, Fung KY, Head R. Nutrigenetics and nutrigenomics: viewpoints on the current status and applications in nutrition research and practice. J

Nutrigenet Nutrigenomics. 2011;4(2):69-89. doi: 10.1159/000327772. Epub 2011 May 28. PMID: 21625170; PMCID: PMC3121546.

Baxter, L.R. Ernest P. Noble.\Neuropsychopharmacol\43, 2162 (2018). https://doi.org/10.1038/s41386-018-0114-9

Noble EP. Alcoholism and the dopaminergic system: a review. Addict Biol. 1996;1(4):333-48. doi: 10.1080/1355621961000124956. PMID: 12893451.

Avena NM, Rada P, Hoebel BG. Evidence for sugar addiction: behavioral and neurochemical effects of intermittent, excessive sugar intake. Neurosci Biobehav Rev. 2008;32(1):20-39. doi: 10.1016/j.neubiorev.2007.04.019. Epub 2007 May 18. PMID: 17617461; PMCID: PMC2235907.

Srámek P, Simecková M, Janský L, Savlíková J, Vybíral S. Human physiological responses to immersion into water of different temperatures. Eur J Appl Physiol. 2000 Mar;81(5):436-42. doi: 10.1007/s004210050065. PMID: 10751106.

Chen C, Chen C, Moyzis R, Stern H, He Q, Li H, Li J, Zhu B, Dong Q. Contributions of dopamine-related genes and environmental factors to highly sensitive personality: a multi-step neuronal system-level approach. PLoS One. 2011;6(7):e21636. doi: 10.1371/journal.pone.0021636. Epub 2011 Jul 13. PMID: 21765900; PMCID: PMC3135587.

Food Addiction definition. Accessed 2024:
https://www.semanticscholar.org/paper/Food-Addiction-A-Disorder-in-Search-of-Diagnostic-Vasiliu-Davila/89e9d8c4c745e0a19bfd3018d656d1f41e640cdb

DRD2

Beaulieu JM, Gainetdinov RR. The physiology, signaling, and pharmacology of dopamine receptors. Pharmacol Rev. 2011 Mar;63(1):182-217. doi: 10.1124/pr.110.002642. Epub 2011 Feb 8. PMID: 21303898.

Missale C, Nash SR, Robinson SW, Jaber M, Caron MG. Dopamine receptors: from structure to function. Physiol Rev. 1998 Jan;78(1):189-225. doi: 10.1152/physrev.1998.78.1.189. PMID: 9457173.

Bari A, Robbins TW. Inhibition and impulsivity: behavioral and neural basis of response control. Prog Neurobiol. 2013 Sep;108:44-79. doi: 10.1016/j.pneurobio.2013.06.005. Epub 2013 Jul 13. PMID: 23856628.

Noble EP. D2 dopamine receptor gene in psychiatric and neurologic disorders and its phenotypes. Am J Med Genet B Neuropsychiatr Genet. 2003 Jan 1;116B(1):103-25. doi: 10.1002/ajmg.b.10005. PMID: 12497624.

Aliasghari F, Nazm SA, Yasari S, Mahdavi R, Bonyadi M. Associations of the ANKK1 and DRD2 gene polymorphisms with overweight, obesity and hedonic hunger among women from the Northwest of Iran [published online ahead of print, 2020 Feb 4]. Eat Weight Disord.2020; doi:10.1007/s40519-020-00851-5Roth

MC4R

Arrizabalaga, M., Larrarte, E., Margareto, J., Maldonado-Martín, S., Barrenechea, L., & Labayen, I. (2014). Preliminary findings on the influence of FTO rs9939609 and MC4R rs17782313 polymorphisms on resting energy expenditure, leptin and thyrotropin levels in obese non-morbid premenopausal women. Journal of physiology and biochemistry, 70(1), 255-262.

Acosta, A., Camilleri, M., Shin, A., Carlson, P., Burton, D., O'Neill, J., Zinsmeister, A. R. (2014). Association of melanocortin 4 receptor gene variation with satiation and gastric emptying in overweight and obese adults. Genes & nutrition, 9(2), 1-7.

MAOA

Function of MAOA gene. Accessed 2024: https://medlineplus.gov/genetics/gene/maoa/

Bortolato M, Chen K, Godar SC, Chen G, Wu W, Rebrin I, Farrell MR, Scott AL, Wellman CL, Shih JC. Social deficits and perseverative behaviors, but not overt aggression, in MAO-A hypomorphic mice. Neuropsychopharmacology. 2011 Dec;36(13):2674-88. doi: 10.1038/npp.2011.157. Epub 2011 Aug 10. PMID: 21832987; PMCID: PMC3230491.
Pizzinat N, Copin N, Vindis C, Parini A, Cambon C. Reactive oxygen species production by monoamine oxidases in intact cells. Naunyn Schmiedebergs Arch Pharmacol. 1999 May;359(5):428-31. doi: 10.1007/pl00005371. PMID: 10498294.

Cases O, Seif I, Grimsby J, Gaspar P, Chen K, Pournin S, Müller U, Aguet M, Babinet C, Shih JC, et al. Aggressive behavior and altered amounts of brain serotonin and norepinephrine in mice lacking MAOA. Science. 1995 Jun 23;268(5218):1763-6. doi: 10.1126/science.7792602. PMID: 7792602; PMCID: PMC2844866.

Wang M, Li H, Deater-Deckard K, Zhang W. Interacting Effect of Catechol-O-Methyltransferase (COMT) and Monoamine Oxidase A (MAOA) Gene Polymorphisms, and Stressful Life Events on Aggressive Behavior in Chinese Male Adolescents. Front Psychol. 2018 Jul 3;9:1079. doi: 10.3389/fpsyg.2018.01079. PMID: 30018578; PMCID: PMC6037980.

Camarena B, Santiago H, Aguilar A, Ruvinskis E, González-Barranco J, Nicolini H. Family-based association study between the monoamine oxidase A gene and obesity: implications for psychopharmacogenetic studies. Neuropsychobiology. 2004;49(3):126-9. doi: 10.1159/000076720. PMID: 15034227.

Chapter 7

Hansen M, Kennedy BK. Does Longer Lifespan Mean Longer Healthspan? Trends Cell Biol. 2016 Aug;26(8):565-568. doi: 10.1016/j.tcb.2016.05.002. Epub 2016 May 27. PMID: 27238421; PMCID: PMC4969078.

Clear, James. Atomic Habits; An Easy and Proven Way to Build Good Habits and Break Bad Ones (2018) ISBN: 9781847941831
Duhigg, C. The Power of Habit: Why We Do What We Do in Life and Business (2014); ISBN: 081298160X

Nestor, James, Breath: The New Science of a Lost Art, (2020); ISBN: 0735213615 p.206.

Chaix R, Alvarez-López MJ, Fagny M, Lemee L, Regnault B, Davidson RJ, Lutz A, Kaliman P. Epigenetic clock analysis in long-term meditators. Psychoneuroendocrinology. 2017 Nov;85:210-214. doi:10.1016/j.psyneuen.2017.08.016.

Yuhong Dong, Chian-Feng Huang, Jim Liao, Alex Chih-Yu Chen, Jason G. Liu, and Kai-Hsiung Hsu. An observational cohort study on terminal cancer survivors practicing falun gong (FLG) in China. 2016. Journal of Clinical Oncology. DOI:10.1200/JCO.2016.34.15_suppl.e21568 https://ascopubs.org/doi/abs/10.1200/JCO.2016.34.15_suppl.e21568

Li QZ, Li P, Garcia GE, Johnson RJ, Feng L. Genomic profiling of neutrophil transcripts in Asian Qigong practitioners: a pilot study in gene regulation by mind-body interaction. J Altern Complement Med. 2005 Feb;11(1):29-39. doi: 10.1089/acm.2005.11.29. PMID: 15750361.

Trey, Margaret & West-Olatunji, Cirecie. 2020. Use of Falun Gong to Address Traumatic Stress among Marginalized Clients. DOI: 10.5772/intechopen.93301

Bendig BW, Shapiro D, Zaidel E. Group differences between practitioners and novices in hemispheric processing of attention and emotion before and after a session of Falun Gong qigong. Brain and Cognition. 2020;138:105494
Pascoe MC, Thompson DR, Jenkins ZM, et al. Mindfulness mediates the physiological markers of stress: systematic review and meta-analysis. *Journal of Psychiatric Research*. 2017;95:156-178.

Lindberg DA. Integrative review of research related to meditation, spirituality, and the elderly. Geriatr Nurs. 2005 Nov-Dec;26(6):372-7. doi: 10.1016/j.gerinurse.2005.09.013. PMID: 16373182.

Koenig HG. Religion, spirituality, and health: the research and clinical implications. ISRN Psychiatry. 2012 Dec 16;2012:278730. doi: 10.5402/2012/278730. PMID: 23762764; PMCID: PMC3671693.

Emmons, R., The Gratitude Project: How the Science of Thankfulness Can Rewire Our Brains for Resilience, Optimism, and the Greater Good. Paperback 9781684034611. Published: September 2020.

Measuring Compassion in the Body. Accessed 2024:
https://greatergood.berkeley.edu/article/item/measuring_compassion_in_the_body

Cregg, D.R., Cheavens, J.S. Gratitude Interventions: Effective Self-help? A Meta-analysis of the Impact on Symptoms of Depression and Anxiety. *J Happiness Stud* 22, 413–445 (2021). https://doi.org/10.1007/s10902-020-00236-6

Peter A. Coventry, Jennifer V.E. Brown, Jodi Pervin, Sally Brabyn, Rachel Pateman, Josefien Breedvelt, Simon Gilbody, Rachel Stancliffe, Rosemary McEachan, PiranC.L. White. Nature-based outdoor activities for mental and physical health: Systematic review and meta-analysis, SSM - Population Health, Volume 16, 2021,100934, ISSN 2352-8273, https://doi.org/10.1016/j.ssmph.2021.100934.
White, M.P., Alcock, I., Grellier, J. *et al.* Spending at least 120 minutes a week in nature is associated with good health and wellbeing. *Sci Rep* 9, 7730. 2019. https://doi.org/10.1038/s41598-019-44097-3

Lieberman MD, Eisenberger NI, Crockett MJ, Tom SM, Pfeifer JH, Way BM. Putting feelings into words: affect labeling disrupts amygdala activity in response to affective stimuli. Psychol Sci. 2007 May;18(5):421-8. doi: 10.1111/j.1467-9280.2007.01916.x. PMID: 17576282.

Wang, J., Mann, F., Lloyd-Evans, B. *et al.* Associations between loneliness and perceived social support and outcomes of mental health problems: a systematic review. *BMC Psychiatry* 18, 156 (2018). https://doi.org/10.1186/s12888-018-1736-5

The Achieving Society. David McClelland, 1961. Accessed 2024: https://psychology.fas.harvard.edu/people/david-mcclelland
Alexander BK, Beyerstein BL, Hadaway BF, Coombs RB. Effect of Early and later colony housing on oral ingestion of morphine in rats. *Pharmacol Biochem Behav.* 1981;15:571-576.

Love and longevity: A Social Dependency Hypothesis (2021) Alexander J.Horna C. Sue Carter-bhttps://doi.org/10.1016/j.cpnec.2021.100088

Wu Youyou 1 2, David Stillwell 3, H Andrew Schwartz 4, Michal Kosinski 5
Birds of a Feather Do Flock Together
Psychol Sci. 2017 Mar;28(3):403. doi: 10.1177/0956797617697667.PMID: 28287052

Allen, Summer. 2018. The Science of Gratitude. UC Berkeley: John Templeton Foundation. Accessed 2024: https://ggsc.berkeley.edu/images/uploads/GGSC-JTF_White_Paper-Gratitude-FINAL.pdf

Chapter 8

Wang DD, Li Y, Bhupathiraju SN, Rosner BA, Sun Q, Giovannucci EL, Rimm EB, Manson JE, Willett WC, Stampfer MJ, Hu FB. Fruit and Vegetable Intake and Mortality: Results From 2 Prospective Cohort Studies of US Men and Women and a Meta-Analysis of 26 Cohort Studies. Circulation. 2021 Apr 27;143(17):1642-1654. doi: 10.1161/CIRCULATION AHA.120.048996. Epub 2021 Mar 1. PMID: 33641343; PMCID: PMC8084888.

Christine A. Houghton, Robert G. Fassett, and Jeff S. Coombes
Sulforaphane and Other Nutrigenomic Nrf2 Activators: Can the Clinician's Expectation Be Matched by the Reality? (2016) Oxid Med Cell Longev. 2016: 7857186. doi: 10.1155/2016/7857186 https://www.ncbi.nlm.nih.gov/pmc/articles/PMC4736808/

Walker, AF, Marakis, G, Christie, S & Byng, M 2003, 'Mg citrate found more bioavailable than other Mg preparations in a randomised, double-blind study', Magnesium Research, vol. 16, no. 3, pp. 183-91.

Owen GN, Parnell H, De Bruin EA, Rycroft JA. The combined effects of L-theanine and caffeine on cognitive performance and mood. Nutr Neurosci. 2008 Aug;11(4):193-8. doi: 10.1179/147683008X301513. PMID: 18681988.
Kakuda T. Neuroprotective effects of theanine and its preventive effects on cognitive dysfunction. Pharmacol Res. 2011;64(2):162-168.

Omega 3s improve Gut Health: *Scientific Reports, 2017;*7:11079

Apple Cider Vinegar timing for blood sugar & digestive (HCL benefits)
Budak, NH et al (2014) Functional properties of vinegar. Journal of Food Science, 79:5

Johnston CS, Steplewska I, Long CA, Harris LN, Ryals RH. Examination of the antiglycemic properties of vinegar in healthy adults. Ann Nutr Metab. 2010;56(1):74-9. doi: 10.1159/000272133. PMID: 20068289.
Jiang T, Gao X, Wu C, Tian F, Lei Q, Bi J, Xie B, Wang HY, Chen S, Wang X. Apple-Derived Pectin Modulates Gut Microbiota, Improves Gut Barrier Function, and Attenuates Metabolic Endotoxemia in Rats with Diet-Induced Obesity. Nutrients. 2016 Feb 29;8(3):126. doi: 10.3390/nu8030126. PMID: 26938554; PMCID: PMC4808856.

Bruins, M. J., Mugambi, G., Verkaik-Kloosterman, J., Hoekstra, J., Kraemer, K., Osendarp, S., Melse-Boonstra, A., Gallagher, A. M., & Verhagen, H. (2015). "Addressing the risk of inadequate and excessive micronutrient intakes: traditional versus new approaches to setting adequate and safe micronutrient levels in foods". *Food & nutrition research*, 59, 26020.

ACKNOWLEDGEMENTS

Writing this book was a much bigger challenge than I had ever imagined.

As a lifelong learner, I've gained many insights from numerous health and behaviour experts over many years. Many I have referenced throughout this book, though I can't remember them all.

I am eternally grateful for the help and suggestions I received from colleagues and friends in putting this all together.

Special thanks to Kelly Irving. The support and connections I made within her author community were crucial to my progress.

Thanks to input from my wise friends and early readers Mark, Marleen, Richard, Wilma, Louise M, Louise S and Vlad for encouraging me when I most needed it. Your suggestions all helped shape this book.

The word-sculpting skills of Lu Sexton and Alan Ferris helped remove the less useful content and give clarity to my message. Special thanks to Arjan Van Woensel for the beautiful cover and interior formatting.

My gratitude extends to all my patients, who remind me why I do this work. Your search for safe and effective natural treatments drives my continuous learning. You have accompanied me down this path and I appreciate every one of you.

Thank you to my grandparents and parents for your enduring love and acceptance of who I am. To my dear sister and best friend, Michelle Genrich, I treasure your unwavering support and love.

To my teenage son, Ashton, you are my inspiration every day. I love you dearly and appreciate the many ways you show me where I need to grow to be a better parent every day.

To my spiritual teacher, Mr. Li Hongzhi. Thank you for giving me hope during those darkest times. Your teachings lift my outlook on life and provide an inner strength to resolve challenges. Thank you for the boundless compassion and wisdom you've provided me and many others.

To you, dear reader, thank you for your trust and investment. Your time is precious and I truly hope reading this makes a difference in your life.

ABOUT THE AUTHOR

Sheridan Genrich, BHSc. is a clinical nutritionist and naturopath whose consulting practice since 2009 has specialised in helping people who struggle with digestive discomfort, addictions, sleep, and mood disturbances.

During her complementary medicine degree at university, Sheridan developed a passion for understanding behavioural neuroscience and gut-brain imbalances. Since then she has completed extensive post-graduate certifications in nutrigenomics, polyvagal theory in trauma and other nutritional healing approaches using the 'food first' principles.

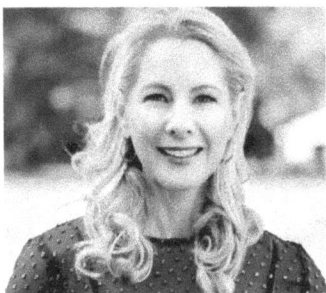

As a highly sensitive person who has learned to thrive again after years of extraordinary adversity, Sheridan is confident that anyone can unlock their innate potential and heal with the right tools and support. She truly believes in using ancestral approaches that are both personalised and aligned with nature's rhythms.

Originally from Australia, she lived in England for several years and recently moved to the United States. When Sheridan is not at work, she loves taking long walks, listening to music, podcasts or books, working out, relaxing in water and being creative in the kitchen.

www.ingramcontent.com/pod-product-compliance
Lightning Source LLC
Chambersburg PA
CBHW011829020426
42334CB00027B/2990